American Special Education

PETER LANG
New York • Washington, D.C./Baltimore • Bern
Frankfurt am Main • Berlin • Brussels • Vienna • Oxford

Gerard Giordano

American Special Education

A History of Early Political Advocacy

PETER LANG
New York • Washington, D.C./Baltimore • Bern
Frankfurt am Main • Berlin • Brussels • Vienna • Oxford

Library of Congress Cataloging-in-Publication Data

Giordano, Gerard.
American special education: a history of early political advocacy /
Gerard Giordano.
p. cm.
Includes bibliographical references and index.
1. Special education—United States. I. Title.
LC3981.G5   371.90973—dc22   2006022445
ISBN 978-0-8204-8695-6

Bibliographic information published by **Die Deutsche Bibliothek**.
Die Deutsche Bibliothek lists this publication in the "Deutsche
Nationalbibliografie"; detailed bibliographic data is available
on the Internet at http://dnb.ddb.de/.

Cover design by Lisa Barfield

The paper in this book meets the guidelines for permanence and durability
of the Committee on Production Guidelines for Book Longevity
of the Council of Library Resources.

© 2007 Peter Lang Publishing, Inc., New York
29 Broadway, 18th floor, New York, NY 10006
www.peterlang.com

Printed in the United States of America

Contents

Preface

It is always an illuminating procedure to trace the path along which we have come, to become acquainted with the historical forces that are driving us, and their directions, because after all we have to conquer, not by opposing these forces, but by conforming to them.

—*White, 1949*

Pedagogy, Politics, and History

During the 1990s, I had been studying the different ways in which children had been taught to read. Although I had intended to limit my studies to twentieth-century practices, I became interested in the instructional techniques and materials of the preceding era. After examining the written advice that early scholars had provided, I discerned ways in which they clearly had attempted to influence educational practices. However, I wondered about their motives. They obviously had been concerned about contemporary teachers and students. Had they also been concerned about future teachers and students?

Before I could investigate this matter, I had to address some procedural matters. For example, I had to locate a classification scheme with which to catalogue nineteenth-century literacy practices. To my disappointment, I was unable to find an appropriate scheme from the nineteenth century. Therefore I eclectically sampled twentieth-century practices. I used this information to assemble an expedient scheme, which I then adapted for nineteenth-century educational practices (Giordano, 2000). In the process of assembling the expedient scheme, I reviewed the distinctive philosophies and peculiar pedagogies of twentieth-century scholars. In spite of their idiosyncrasies, all of the scholars had deferred to three factors: the language skills of learners, the content of instructional materials, and the pedagogical system with which instruction had been organized. Some twentieth-century literacy scholars also paid attention to distinctive instructional technologies. After I had incorporated the first three factors into an expedient taxonomy, I decided that the addition of the technological factor would enhance its usefulness.

Even though they may have embraced common pedagogical elements, the twentieth-century academicians placed differential emphases upon them. For example, some of them had prioritized decoding skills. Believing that phonics would enable students to "sound out" unfamiliar words, they insisted that reading approaches reinforce phonics. Even the most doctrinaire partisans had not wished to categorically exclude the language skills of students or the content of instructional materials. Nonetheless, their insistence on a phonics-centered regimen effectively deemphasized the content of passages and the students' own language.

The proponents of literature-based approaches had their own priorities. Wishing to emphasize the content of books, they demanded that all instructional materials contain substantive content. They believed that this feature would entice students. The proponents of literature-based approaches did not wish to prevent instructors from using decoding drills or language-based exercises. However, they did believe that the most sensible approach would focus students' attention on the content of books.

The proponents of decoding skills and the proponents of literature-based skills had emphasized different aspects of literacy instruction. Nonetheless, the members of both groups agreed that they should stress only a single dimension of the reading program. Following this pattern, the advocates of language-based instruction decided to prioritize oral language. In fact, they recommended that oral-language exercises accompany all reading instruction.

The proponents of technology-based instruction formed the fourth literacy faction. They demonstrated strategic behaviors that replicated those of the other three groups. When they had to choose a preeminent feature of instruction, they selected technology. Quite understandably, their philosophical outlook convinced them that pedagogical technology would substantively influence students who were learning to read.

When I had begun my investigation of literacy education, I had wondered whether the pioneers in this field had resolved to affect future educational practices. I was unable to answer this precise question. However, the early scholars had ample opportunities to visualize the literacy practices that their pedagogical heirs would employ. More notably, they had developed the prototypes for the subsequent practices. They had fully implemented the skills-based, language-based, and literature-based approaches. Although they had not used the technology-based approach widely, they understood it well enough to envisage subsequent developments. Their approaches had exhibited the essential features of twentieth-century instruction.

Many of the early literacy educators had advocated a single approach to instruction. They had written editorials, research reports, and monographs in which they praised the particular approach that they had selected. The academicians from other fields had engaged in comparable practices. In the middle of the twentieth century, Saveth (1952) underscored the feuding among those professors who endorsed selective approaches to social studies instruction. He conceded that the professors had been able to publish their diatribes only in "dull" academic monographs. Nonetheless, Saveth was convinced that the professors still had been able to politically indoctrinate citizens. He claimed that this ideological dissemination had been extremely effective because of the professors' access to legions of teachers. These teachers subsequently had influenced the elementary-school or high-school students who were in their own classes.

Saveth (1952) believed that the instructional interactions of professors, teachers, and public-school students revealed the complex manner in which the educational system could affect national events. An ardent political conservative, Saveth was especially upset by those professors and public-school teachers who had advanced the political interests of the Democratic Party. He was convinced that these liberal activists had been able to influence the outcomes of national elections. Saveth took some solace in the fact that conservative educators recently had taken measures to reverse the liberal educators' "distorted treatments" of American history and current events. He noted that these intellectual countermeasures constituted "significant contributions toward the creation of that conservative synthesis which is needed to challenge Fair Deal influence in historical writing, [*sic*] and at the polls as well" (p. 118).

Saveth (1952) was not the only person with strong convictions about the ways in which scholars could affect educational trends and national issues. Although they were concerned about special educators rather than social studies educators, Frampton and Rowell (1938) had shared some of Saveth's assumptions. In their history of special education, they had revealed their view about the power that special education scholars could wield.

> [Our book] is devoted to revealing the growth, through the ages, of the care and education of the handicapped, with stress upon those things in the past which have influenced the present or may influence the future either positively or negatively. Since great personages rather than momentous events have been the outstanding influences in this history, the material has been organized generally on the basis of the Great Man Theory. (p. xi)

Frampton and Rowell (1938) had indicated that they subscribed to the "Great Man Theory." This theory assumed that individual leaders could have an immense impact on society. Frampton and Rowell were professors at Teachers College, which had attracted some of the most politically liberal faculty members of that period. Despite their own theoretical convictions, Frampton and Rowell recognized that most of their peers at Teachers College had rejected "the Great Man Theory." This awareness may have influenced them when they pledged to follow their 1938 treatise with a book that represented a philosophically different perspective. Frampton and Rowell assured readers that their next book would represent politically progressive social views. They explained that it would "deal specifically with relevant and pertinent problems, attitudes, and trends . . . of the present time, with some consideration of the future" (p. xi).

In a study that they conducted more than 60 years after the publication of the Frampton and Rowell book, a group of educational researchers ("Classic Articles," 2004) relied again on the "Great Man Theory." These researchers tried to identify those scholars who had written the reports that had caused the most significant impact on the field of special education. However, they were frustrated. After conducting their research, they failed to detect any "consensus regarding which articles have shaped the field of special education" (p. 79).

After I had completed my own research, I questioned whether the "Great Man Theory" was relevant to the history of literacy education. I had not discerned educators who had changed the course of society. I had not discerned any who had changed the course of national political movements. I had not detected any who clearly had changed the pedagogy that prevailed in the schools. To the contrary, it seemed that social and political movements had affected the popularity of educational practices and the scholars who had espoused those practices.

Impressed by the degree to which politics had influenced literacy education, I wondered about the ways in which politics might have influenced other educational trends. Therefore, I followed my study of literacy with three specialized investigations. I examined the use of twentieth-century textbooks, the changes that had transpired in wartime schools, and the expansion of scholastic testing. In these studies (Giordano, 2003; 2004; 2005), I concentrated my attention on the interplay of prevalent and emerging attitudes toward education. However, I also examined interconnected attitudes toward race, religion, gender, employment, immigration, economic growth, military preparedness, and international security.

My follow-up studies gave me the opportunity to look for ways in which eminent scholars had influenced the schools. They also gave me the chance to search for ways in which scholars had used the shifting zeitgeist to advance some ulterior cause.

With regard to the initial opportunity, I failed to discern compelling examples of ways in which eminent scholars had influenced the schools. However, I was able to detect multiple examples of politically hardnosed and preeminently pragmatic educators who at first had supported but then later abandoned specific initiatives. Early twentieth-century progressive educators had provided compelling examples of such pragmatic behaviors.

The progressive educators had designed a pedagogical approach to complement their liberal political platform. However, they were unprepared for the objections that the World War I conservatives raised. The conservatives faulted the progressive educators for failing to nurture critical values and skills. They claimed that this educational lapse had imperiled the nation's economic prosperity and military security. Once they realized that a large segment of the wartime public agreed with the conservatives, the progressive educators reversed their original stance toward the politicization of educational initiatives. The conservatives, who were as pragmatic as the progressive educators, were surprised by the success of their political campaign. As a result, they politicized additional educational initiatives.

Liberals and conservatives continued to contest educational issues. They sparred over trivial and fundamental issues. In fact, different factions of liberals sometimes disagreed with each other about whether a particular issue was trivial or fundamental. This type of disagreement was apparent in the ways that they reacted to textbooks. Most liberals believed that textbooks inhibited the creativity of teachers, suppressed the imagination of learners, and discouraged individualized education. In spite of these views, moderate liberals did not consider textbooks to be fundamental determinants of effective schooling. Therefore they were willing to deal with these difficulties by modifying textbooks. Unlike their moderate colleagues, liberal extremists saw textbooks as a substantive issue. Based on this conviction, they categorically opposed any use of textbooks. As for the conservatives, they generally supported textbooks. Although they disagreed with the moderate liberals, they decided to accommodate their demands (Giordano, 2003). As a result, the conservatives were able to deflect the attack on textbooks from extremist liberals. They were successful in numerous other encounters, especially during World War I, World War II, and the cold war (Giordano, 2004). They also were victorious in the long battle over educational testing (Giordano, 2005).

Twentieth-century liberals won their own share of educational confrontations. They reformulated the ways in which religion, gender, and ethnicity were depicted in classrooms (Giordano, 2003). They modified the use of assessment and instructional materials (Giordano, 2005). Although numerous initiatives attracted support from the liberals, two of them were truly monumental. One of these was the drive to help students from racial minority groups. The other was the drive to aid students with disabilities.

Educating Individuals With Disabilities

The nineteenth- and early twentieth-century educational reformers were pragmatists. They sometimes made appeals to liberals and at other times to conservatives. Historically, each of these political groups had opposed those initiatives that their rivals had endorsed. Nonetheless, the liberals and conservatives occasionally had collaborated. For example, some persons from both groups had cooperated in order to sustain the use of textbooks in the schools. Some persons from both groups also had cooperated to address the enduring problems of the students from racial minority groups.

During the 1960s, liberals and conservatives again cooperated. Both groups were attempting to resolve some of the centuries-long educational problems that individuals with disabilities had faced. The liberals and conservatives recognized that cooperation would increase their political might. As one would expect, persons with disabilities and their families were attracted to this alliance. Caregivers, instructors, physicians, and individuals who interacted directly with disabled persons also were attracted. Many scientists, lawyers, community leaders, judges, businesspersons, journalists, and social activists joined them.

The members of the 1960s coalition viewed children with disabilities from a new and distinctive perspective. Early scholars had recognized that genetic and medical handicaps could impair vision, hearing, oral communication, language, mobility, and mental operations. They also had recognized many of the ways in which these conditions could restrict learning. However, the early scholars had underestimated the influence of academic, social, and emotional factors on learning. The members of the new coalition began to view children with disabilities in a comprehensive manner; they also began to explore the pedagogical and political implications of that perspective.

Many persons joined the movement to help special learners. All of them were helpful. Nonetheless, parents may have played the most important role. They adjured federal lawmakers to enact laws to define and protect the rights of their children. They insisted that the lawmakers disseminate, regulate, and finance special education. While continuing to call attention to those disabilities that had been recognized historically, they simultaneously raised awareness about little-known disabilities. For example, they publicized the problems of intelligent students who were unable to read, write, or calculate. They demonstrated that even extraordinary talented students could exhibit subtle types of disabilities.

From the beginning, political forces shaped American education. Comparable forces affected special education. They influenced the debates about the nature, scope, and etiology of disabilities. They enabled community-based care and instruction to emerge. They helped popularize novel assessment approaches and controversial learning techniques. They promoted a perspective that depicted students with disabilities as productive, independent, self-fulfilled, and respected.

Acknowledgment

I cannot express sufficient gratitude to my extraordinarily talented research assistant, Renee Wyden. Without her collaboration, this book would not have been written.

List of Illustrations

1

Humanitarian and Moral Issues

As in other works of philanthropy, so in [the movement to educate persons with disabilities], other laborers were ready at once to enter into the harvest.
—Brockett, 1855

Scholars and educators initially placed few restrictions on expressions such as *idiocy*, *feeblemindedness*, and *backwardness*. Although they later saw the need to employ these terms with precision, they could not agree about fundamental issues. For example, they disagreed about the extent to which environmental and genetic factors influenced disabilities. They also disagreed about the way to treat disabled persons. Those who viewed disabled persons as dangerous supported asylum-based care. Those who believed that the danger was minimal recommended community-based care. Even though members of the public were distressed at the many questions that remained unresolved, they showed progressively greater tolerance to persons with disabilities. They eventually resolved to provide educational opportunities to them.

Searching for Terminology

Nineteenth-century contemporaries easily could discern the ways in which large political movements were affecting society. These movements substantively altered legal systems, economies, governments, and national boundaries. In addition to changing the global dimensions of society, the movements transformed quotidian aspects of individual lives. They influenced employment, military duty, safety, social status, political rights, and property.

The large political movements of the nineteenth century affected society directly. They also affected many individuals directly. However, the influence of these movements was compounded through the derivative events that they stimulated. Sometimes these derivative events, even though they involved relatively few persons and attracted only a modest amount of attention, had a pervasive impact. As with pebbles tossed into a pond, they created ripples that changed the water's entire surface.

When special education was tossed into the pond of nineteenth-century society, few observers discerned a splash. In fact, few of them discerned any ripples. Brockett (1855) was an exception. He chronicled some of the experiments that had affected persons with disabilities. These small-scale but critically important experiments had been initiated during the early part of the nineteenth century. Brockett described this as the era when "the condition of the idiot began to attract the attention of the humane" (p. 593).

Brockett (1855) was struck by the remarkable achievements of two pioneers in the field of special education. One of these persons was Jean-Marc Itard. Brockett was impressed with the manner in which Itard had analyzed and then helped a young man who became known as the "Savage of Aveyron." Although he was amazed by Itard's educational expertise, Brockett was equally impressed with Itard's ability to use educational incidents as pretexts for changing societal attitudes. Brockett judged that Itard had influenced the way in which contemporary scholars, professionals, and the general public viewed persons with disabilities.

Brockett (1855) identified Edward Seguin as the other scholar who had made a great impression on him. Brockett respected Seguin, who was one of Itard's pupils, for initiating "the private instruction of idiots" (p. 593). Brockett pointed out that Seguin had used "inextinguishable love for his race, indomitable perseverance, a highly cultivated intellect, and a rare degree of executive talent" to rescue many "hapless creatures . . . from the doom of a life of utter vacuity" (p. 593). Writing more than half of a century later, Van Sickle, Witmer, and Ayres, (1911) indicated that they and many other scholars continued to admire Seguin. They eulogized his work as "a model for the countries of the civilized world" (p. 11).

Brockett (1855) had entitled his nineteenth-century report *Idiots and Institutions for Their Training*. Even though he used the term *idiocy* throughout his book, Brockett never defined it. Contemporary British scholars showed the same disregard for definitions. Duncan (1866) later concluded that these scholars had not defined *idiocy*, or other expressions such as *imbecility* and *feeblemindedness*, because they were sure that these terms conveyed "a meaning readily understood, and it may appear useless to analyse [*sic*] the mental condition thereby represented" (p. 1). Disagreeing with earlier scholars, Duncan wrote that "it is necessary to separate many of the classes into which the cases [of persons with disabilities] may be divided, for the purpose of training" (p. 1).

Duncan (1866) had insisted that scholars devise precise definitions for the terms they were employing. Several years later, William Ireland (1877) sided with him. Ireland was an extremely influential British scientist and educator. Like Duncan, he speculated about the reason that British scholars had been hesitant to offer a definition of idiocy. Ireland thought they had made this omission primarily because they judged idiocy to be "a popular, [*sic*] and not a scientific term" (p. 1). Ireland added that "the condition which it signifies is easily recognizable, and the word idiocy, or some other equivalent term, is to be found in the languages of all civilized nations" (p. 1). In spite these exculpatory circumstances, Ireland agreed with Duncan about the need to establish a common context for terms that were being used with increasing frequency. As for the term *idiot*, Ireland pointed out that the authorities who had managed the 1870 American census had used this term to classify 24,395 persons. However, he had no sooner reported this observation than he discredited it. Ireland observed that "none of those specially acquainted with the subject of idiocy in America have much faith in the result of the general census of idiots in the United States" (p. 14).

Although few educators had defined the terms they were using, most of them had tried to clarify them through case studies. To help readers conceptualize the physical correlates of disabilities, they supplemented their case studies with photographs or artists' illustrations. Ireland (1877) included the illustrations in Figure 1.1 in a nineteenth-century textbook. Figure 1.2 is a table that Ireland placed in the same textbook. Ireland had devised the table in order to provide details of

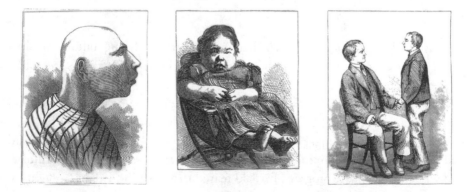

Figure 1.1. Early Scholars Typically Included Illustrations of Persons with Disabilities within their Books.

	CERRETTI.								
	NICOLA. Age 21			SERAFINO. Age 13			GIOVANNI. Age. 10		
	Metres.	Inches.		Metres.	Inches.		Metres.	Inches.	
Height	1·65 =	65		1·35 =	53		1·17 =	46	
	Kilogrammes.			Kilogrammes.			Kilogrammes.		
Weight	56·500			34·00			24·00		
	Mill.	About in.	ls.	Mill.	About in.	ls.	Mill.	About in.	ls.
Fore-head. Curves. { Circumference . .	450 =	17	8	420 =	16	6	410 =	16	2
Antero-posterior . .	240 =	9	5	260 =	10	3	250 =	9	10
Biauricular . .	220 =	8	8	210 =	8	2	220 =	8	8
Breadth . .	100 =	4	0	150 =	5	11	150 =	5	11
Height . .	200 =	7	11	300 =	11	10	200 =	7	11
Diameters. { Longitudinal . .	148 =	5	9	145 =	5	9	140 =	5	6
Transverse . .	122 =	4	9	120 =	4	8	110 =	4	3
Bimastoid . .	120 =	4	8	110 =	4	3	100 =	4	8
Bizygomatic . .	130 =	5	2	103 =	4	0	98 =	3	9
Fronto-mental . .	157 =	6	2	162 =	6	4	130 =	5	2
Occipito-mental . .	200 =	7	11	186 =	7	3	175 =	6	10
Ears. { Length . .	60 =	2	4	48 =	1	9	54 =	2	2
Breadth . .	34 =	1	3	30 =	1	2	30 =	1	2
Length of arm . .	330 =	13		300 =	11	9	210 =	8	2
,, forearm . .	380 =	15		230 =	9	1	165 =	6	6
,, hands . .	190 =	7	6	180 =	7	2	111 =	4	4
,, thigh . .	510 =	20	1	370 =	14	7	290 =	11	4
,, leg below the knee	410 =	16		335 =	13	9	240 =	9	4
,, foot . .	265 =	10	2	230 =	9	1	200 =	7	11
,, calf . .	320 =	12	6	250 =	9	10	210 =	8	3
Distance of auditory meatus to the chin	170 =	6	8	130 =	5	2	140 =	5	6
Distance of do. to bregma .	160 =	6	4	150 =	5	11	145 =	5	9
Distance to root of nose .	140 =	5	6	110 =	4	3	105 =	4	1
Distance of the nasal septum from the alveolar margin .	20 =	0	9	25 =	1	0	15 =	0	5
Fronto-orbital angle . .	115°			122°			100°		
Facial angle	68°			70°			72°		
Force of fist	88			48			40		

Figure 1.2. Some Nineteenth-Century Authors Summarized Information about Disabled Persons.

the physical irregularities to which he had been referring. Throughout the first half of the twentieth century, many authors attached these types of pictures and tables to their scholarly materials.

Walter Fernald (1893) was an American educator who was writing at the end of the nineteenth century. Fernald commented on the damage that inaccurate terminology had been causing. He reported that multiple scholars shared his view and had been suggesting definitions of frequently used terms. Although these scholars had wished to facilitate progress, Fernald feared that their individual espousals of idiosyncratic definitions had produced the opposite effect. Jumping into the middle of this academic fray, Fernald called for definitions exhibiting a precise format, specific organization, and clear-cut type of language.

Fernald (1893) wished to demonstrate the type of definition to which he had alluded. He therefore proffered a model definition for the term "feeble-minded." Although this definition may have been intended to serve as a paradigm to Fernald's professional colleagues, it was so stark that it must have made them pause.

> Modern usage has sanctioned the use of the term "feeble-minded" to include all degrees and types of congenital defect, from that of the simply backward boy or girl but little below the normal standard of intelligence to the profound idiot, a helpless, speechless, disgusting burden, with every degree of deficiency between these extremes. (p. 213)

Because of the different ways in which scholars were applying the term "feeble-minded," Fernald (1893) gave his audience a contextualized as well an academic definition. To establish an appropriate context, he identified the types of individuals who were being admitted to educational programs for the "feeble-minded." Fernald confined his remarks to the seven public and two private American schools that were operating specialized programs in 1874. The schools in question had a total enrollment of 1,110 pupils. Fernald cited three factors that had guided the schools' administrators when they had admitted their "feeble-minded" students. One factor was the physical limitation created by inadequate staff, facilities, and operating budgets. A second factor was a lack of knowledge "of the causes, frequency, nature, or varieties of idiocy, or of the principles and methods to be employed in successfully training and caring for this class of persons" (p. 208). The third factor was the general public's "distrust and doubt as to the value of the results to be obtained [from special education]" (p. 208). Given these challenging circumstances, the supervisory personnel at all nine schools had decided to admit only "higher-grade" patients. Fernald reported that the school administrators had made this decision so that could focus their attention on pupils for whom "the resulting improvement and development could be compared with that of normal children" (p. 209).

Writing at the end of the twentieth century, Trent (1998) investigated some of the ways in which special education terminology historically had been used. He specifically examined printed documents that had contained references to individuals with disabilities and that had been distributed during the 1904 World's Fair. Trent noted that the authors of these items had alluded to persons with disabilities as "defectives." Assuming that their audience would understand this term, the authors had not provided an accompanying definition. Nonetheless, they had tried to help their readers better understand the group to which the term "defectives" referred. For example, they had described some of the educational procedures that had been devised for "defectives." They also had described the eugenic interventions that some individuals thought were appropriate for this class of persons. These interventions included institutionalization, sexual sterilization, and deportation. Trent noted that extermination was another intervention.

Just as some groups advocated for the interests of disabled persons, others lobbied against their interests. The general public had to place this conflicting advice in some type of context. Because they lacked definitions, they had to determine to precisely which disabled individuals the different groups were referring. The general public was not alone; most educators, medical personnel, and scholars were confused by the imprecise manner in which terminology was being applied to persons with disabilities. As a consequence, twentieth-century professionals began to demand the precise use of scholarly language. Kuhlmann (1904) was one of the scholars who specifically had referred to the "great need" for "accurate descriptive terminology" (p. 391). Although he recognized the many definitions of disabilities that had been proffered, Kuhlmann protested that "not one of them is uniformly followed by many writers" (p. 391). Kuhlmann concluded that the "unfortunate" habits of scholars and practitioners had "made chaos of much of the literature" (p. 391).

Writing at the beginning of the twentieth century, Kohs (1916) looked back on the historical disputes about terminology. He recognized that many of the early disagreements still had not been resolved. Unlike most of his colleagues, Kohs was not distressed at this situation. He even offered a philosophical rationalization to convince his irate colleagues that they should adopt his calm demeanor.

> Disagreement, in the early development of any field, often makes for progress. Unanimity at that time is inherently conservative, and may frequently lead to stagnation and regression. . . . Difference of opinion is inherent in a growing realm of science. It is therefore no unnecessary defect to find great variance in the interpretation of the facts of any natural phenomenon, especially if some of the aspects are social. The one-hundred years' history of the study and treatment of mental deficiency amply reveals the undercurrent of this progressive tendency. Of late, differences have perhaps increased because of the refinement of general methods by which the feeble-minded may be diagnosed, as a result of attempts to define, examine and report the problem more accurately. Some authorities define mental deficiency one way, [*sic*] others define it some other way. (p. 88)

Kohs had made the preceding observations more than a decade and a half into the twentieth century. Not sharing his upbeat disposition, most of his professional colleagues ignored his advice.

British Scholars Hunt for Scientific Terms

During the nineteenth century and the early part of the twentieth century, scholars were assembling a body of knowledge about special education. Many educators, medical personnel, and members of the public saw immediate and future applications for this knowledge. However, they were confused because so much of this information remained scientifically disorganized. This disorganization was partially the result of the expedient scholastic practices on which teachers had been relying. The efforts to make special education more scientific were blocked by practitioners and theorists who could not agree among themselves about the ways in which they were using fundamental concepts. In a 1904 report, the members of the Royal Commission of Great Britain had tried to solve this problem. This commission's members had employed a clear and accessible style of writing to create definitions that were both scientifically valid and practical. Their approach was evident in the way that they defined a "feeble-minded" person.

> [A feeble-minded person is] one who is capable of making a living under favorable circumstances, but is incapable from mental defect existing from birth or from an early age (a) of competing on equal terms with his normal fellows, or (b) of managing himself and his affairs with ordinary prudence. (Passage from the report of the Royal Commission of Great Britain, 1904, as quoted by Hollingworth, 1922, p. 36)

Crowely (1910) wished to extend definitions beyond the parameters that the Royal Commission had set. Specifically, he wanted definitions to include information about the causes as well as the effects of disabilities. Crowely observed that "the disabilities from which a child may suffer may be either physical or mental, or these two combined" (p. 83). He thought that distinctions of the types that he had introduced were just the beginning points for protracted and complex investigations. Crowely explained that "the great work, then, which lies in front of the educationist [*sic*] concerned with elementary education is to define these various groups [of students with disabilities], and having defined them to pursue the matter to its logical conclusion" (p. 83).

Sherlock (1911), who had been the superintendent of a British asylum, wrote a comprehensive textbook that he entitled *The Feeble-Minded: A Guide to Study and Practice*. Within the preface to his book, Sherlock tried to parse some of the bewildering terminology that had been applied to students with disabilities.

> "Degeneracy" implies the falling from a higher estate, whereas it is the failure to reach the normal one which is the more obvious characteristic. "Amentia" errs in the other

direction. It suggests that the defect observed is entirely due to laggard development; a suggestion which, as will be seen later, is not particularly well founded. Moreover, the term "Amentia" is widely used to denote states of confusional [*sic*] insanity. "Mental Deficiency" is too comprehensive, while "Idiocy" and "Imbecility" are too restricted in the application. One might, perhaps, speak of "Physical Hypertrophy" or utilize the Greek word "$\mu\omega\rho\iota\alpha$," which, whatever it may have meant originally, has now so few associations that any desired signification might be attached to it. On the whole, however, it seems best to follow the lead of a recent Royal Commission and employ the term "Feeble-Mindedness." (pp. vi-vii)

Sherlock had revealed the degree to which the use of definitions in Great Britain remained contentious. Nonetheless, his remark about the need to respect the work of the Royal Commission was an early step toward consensus.

American Scholars Look for Scientific Terms

Barr (1904) had written one of the early twentieth-century histories of special education. In this history, he included an entire chapter on the classification of persons with disabilities. Barr began the chapter with an acknowledgement that "to the student of mental defect the very first requisite is a classification that shall be at once simple and comprehensive, definite and clear" (p. 78). Despite it obvious advantages, the type of classification system to which Barr had referred still had not been devised. He speculated that this failure was the result of "conditions, incident upon diversity of times and nationalities, as well as the differences of bases constituting premises" (p. 78).

European educators had benefited from the highly regarded work of the Royal Commission of Great Britain. Unlike their European colleagues, American educators lacked a common, government-endorsed set of terms with which to distinguish the students who should be eligible for special educational services. As a result, many of them had relied on their own experiences or their professional intuitions. However, the American educators were aware that the public had doubts because the approach that they had designated was unscientific. They therefore tried to demonstrate that their attempts to differentiate students with disabilities from those without disabilities, although these attempts may have been unscientific, had been systematic. As an example, Devereux (1909) described the procedure that was used to admit students from one of Philadelphia's "foreign slum districts" into one of that city's special education classes.

Those children [who were admitted] were reported not only as being stupid, but "queer." It is hard to define exactly what was meant by this term but it did mean that the child to whom it was applied was singled out from the other children. Other children not placed in the class were dull and slow but still normal, while each of these children seemed to have a personality differing from the normal child and also from the purely incorrigible type. . . . While none of the children were monstrosities such as some of those found in institutions, all presented some physical signs of backwardness besides the slow development of mental powers. Of the physiological defects the open mouth, abstracted stare, irregular aimless movements of the limbs, tremors of the body and a general lack of coördination [*sic*] were the common ones. (pp. 45–46)

American school administrators and educators made the best of this confusing situation. Although some of them had confidence in the way that they had been classifying students, most agreed that they needed uniform terminology and procedures. Edson (1906–1907), who was a New York superintendent, addressed this issue forthrightly. He wrote that inaccurate classification and inappropriate teaching had been "responsible for more backwardness on the part of pupils than all other causes combined" (p. 400).

Rogers (1912), who was the Superintendent of the Minnesota School for the Feeble-Minded and Colony for Epileptics, agreed with Edson's criticism. Furthermore, Rogers detected an emerging consensus about the need for uniform terminology. Rogers estimated that "all who for the first time give attention to the literature and treatment of mental defectives are puzzled and confused by the lack of uniformity observed by writers and experienced workers in this field, both in the nomenclature adopted and classifications followed" (p. 135). Even though school personnel may have been distressed by this problem, they were unable to solve it. Rogers lamented that the disputants could not even agree upon "a very satisfactory psychologic [*sic*] classification of scientific value" (p. 135).

Maximillian Groszmann (1913) was another advocate for precise terminology. Like many of his colleagues, he had been struck by the "indefinite and arbitrary use of terms." Groszmann's opinions were important because of his impressive influence on educators and scholars. As to Groszmann's prominence among his contemporaries, the editor of *Educational Foundations* prophesied that "the name of Groszmann will be writ large on the pages of the history of education" (passage from the byline, editor of *Educational Foundations*, 1917, in a report by Groszmann, 1917a, p. 24). After decrying the problems that were caused by the sloppy use of terms, Groszmann assured readers that the use of precise terminology would reduce or eliminate those problems. He then demonstrated a way of developing precise terminology. Groszmann's distinctive solution entailed an elaborate taxonomical diagram. This diagram, which represented an exceptional child, is reproduced in Figure 1.3 (Groszmann, 1913, p. 34).

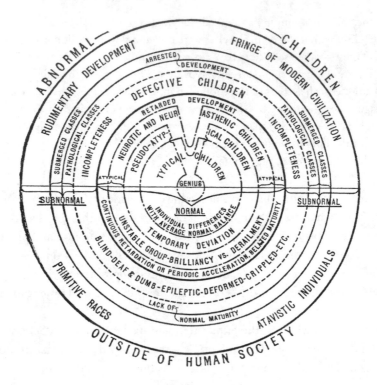

Figure 1.3. Early Twentieth-Century Diagram Depicting the Complex Etiology of Disabilities.

Despite Groszmann's admirable intentions, his esoteric illustration may have created more confusion than it eliminated. Groszmann (1917b) was quite aware that some educators had not been impressed by the way in which he had tried to solve this problem. He advised these critics that they should cease searching for "smooth and inoffensive appellations for children of mentally defective development" (p. vii). Instead, they were to accept his suggestions. The irascible Groszmann was even upset by the persons who had accepted his suggestions but who had done so uncritically. He chastised the members of this group for misappropriating his taxonomical chart in order to make "a euphoric designation for those children who are really abnormal" (p. vii).

Like Groszmann, Gesell (1913) was a prominent scholar during this era. Although he encouraged professionals to carefully classify persons with disabilities, Gesell was not naïve about the difficulty that this change would entail. Wishing to appease his professional colleagues, Gesell attempted to synthesize multiple viewpoints about mental disabilities into a single perspective.

Medically, feeble-mindedness is a permanent, early arrest of the development of the nervous system. . . . Pedagogically, feeble-minded persons are those who cannot be taught to read, write, or cipher, with any marked advantage to themselves or society. Psychologically, feeble-mindedness is a condition of permanent, incurable mental retardation . . . Sociologically, feeble-mindedness is a condition of relative mental incompetence, dating from birth or infancy, which makes it impossible for the individual to get along in the world on equal terms with his normal fellows. (p. 12)

Throughout the early part of the twentieth century, scholars continued to make testimonials about the damage that inaccurate terminology had caused. Within an article entitled "What Constitutes Feeble-Mindedness," Kuhlmann (1915) reviewed disparate definitions of feeblemindedness in order to call "attention to the multiple and discordant standards that are now commonly followed in deciding on the classification of borderline and doubtful cases" (p. 215). O'Shea (1915) made this identical point when he articulated questions of "supreme importance" to teachers and parents. O'Shea's questions emphasized the need to pair terminology and classification procedures with scientific information about the scope, causes, and treatments for disabilities.

When is a child backward? May he be backward in some ways and forward in others? Are children backward by birth, or are they made so by neglect or bad methods of training? What are the signs of backwardness? Is there any way of determining accurately whether or not a given child is permanently arrested? Could the parent and the teacher help an unfortunate child if they could early detect his shortcomings? What part do physical causes play in mental and moral backwardness? Is retardation in childhood and youth even due to the use of stimulants such as tea, coffee, cocoa and alcoholic beverages? What part does food play in determining whether or not a child will be normal intellectually and morally? (p. 1)

O'Shea (1915) had referred to the frustration that parents and teachers were feeling because scholars had not studied special education adequately. Moreover, those scholars who had studied it had relied on undefined terms and concepts. Arthur Holmes (1915), who was the author of the book in which O'Shea had made his critical remarks, failed to follow O'Shea's adjuration. Instead of offering concise, science-based definitions, Holmes filled his book with lengthy case studies. Speaking in his own defense, Holmes explained that he had selected the writing style that he thought would promote an understanding of students with disabilities. That style of writing was "purposely as popular in vein as possible without offending scientific principles or sacrificing exactness in essentials" (p. 5). Holmes felt justified in adopting this approach because "backward children do not present one type of mind, but many types" (p. 58).

The public and many professionals were annoyed at professors and scientists who had refused to write in a concise, accurate, and scientific manner. Bronner (1916) wrote an article in which she explicitly asked, "What do psychiatrists mean by their use of terms in reference to feeble-mindedness?" (p. 32). She responded curtly that "it is difficult to find an adequate answer" (p. 32). After she had identified terms that had been defined clearly by professional organizations in Great Britain and the United States, Bronner berated the many scholars who had ignored those definitions. Bronner stated emphatically that "there is . . . no possible justification for the misuse of these terms" (p. 33).

Writing in the early 1920s, Dealey (1923) was sympathetic to those professionals who had been advocating the use of precise terminology. After she had investigated definitions of the term *problem children*, Dealey noted that the youngsters in this group included "all exceptional children, those above average as well as those below average, children who are 'nervous,' shy ones, sulkers, truants, delinquents, children in any way troublesome, [*sic*] or difficult from the normal, happy child" (pp. 125–126). To demonstrate that this type of problem could be solved, Dealey carefully defined several of the preceding groups.

> By *backward children* are meant those children who repeat in the grade or those doing poor work in the grade in which they are placed. *Nervous children* are those who seem to the teacher extremely restless, or those who make involuntary movements of the hands or of other parts of the body. *Shy children* are those who refrain from joining in the work of the classroom spontaneously, who talk in a low tone, or refuse to answer at all when addressed. (Emphasis in the original text, p. 126)

Mesibov (1976) was aware of the misunderstanding that imprecise terminology had generated during the early part of the twentieth century. He discussed several of the attempts to disentangle that terminology.

> For many years, the words "moron," "imbecile" and "idiot" were used to describe the different levels of mental retardation. The term "moron" referred to an IQ of about 50–70, "imbecile" referred to an IQ of about 30–50, "imbecile" referred to an IQ of about 0–30. Later the term "feebleminded" replaced "moron" in many places, especially Europe. These terms were used until 1954, when the World Health Organization recommended the terms "mild subnormality," "moderate subnormality" and "severe subnormality" to describe the degrees of mental retardation. (p. 25)

Almost 20 years after Mesibov had written the preceding passage, Noll (1995) shared Mesibov's views about the confusion that inaccurate terminology had created.

Noll concluded that "problems of nomenclature and terminology clouded the issue of what actually constituted mental retardation during the first four decades of the twentieth century" (p. 1). Noll had been referring to the historical period from 1900–1940. Writing only 15 years after this period, Frampton and Gall (1955a) had judged that the problems with terminology were still evident. Frampton and Gall concluded that "inaccurate classification of cases" and "much literary license with definitions" remained two of the chief reasons that "the term 'Special Education' today has no concise definition limiting its objectives and field of function" (p. 2).

Concerns About Morality

Shortly after the middle of the twentieth century, Frampton and Gall (1955a; 1955b; 1956) published a three-volume compendium of scientific and practical information about special education. Within the preface to the first book in this set, they noted that services had been available historically to "child and adult deviates." Frampton and Gall reported about five types of services: educational, psychological, social, vocational, and spiritual. They then made a list of the institutions that had provided these services. Even though they placed churches at the head of this list, Frampton and Gall noted that the churches had harmed as well as helped persons with disabilities. Frampton and Gall explained that the historical treatment of individuals with disabilities had been "clouded with superstitions, ideologies, and philosophies conditioned by tribal customs, religious beliefs, economic circumstances, and political experience" (1955a, p. xxii).

Frampton and Gall (1955a) had used the initial statements in their preface to underscore the ways in society's views of morality had influenced special education. Other contributors to Frampton and Gall's encyclopedic publication reaffirmed that view. For example consider the following passage, which detailed the predictable problems that special educators should anticipate when interacting with children from single-parent homes or nontraditional families.

> Progress in the treatment and understanding of problems relating to birth out of wedlock is reflected in the present movement, toward substitution of the term "out of wedlock" for "illegitimacy." The latter, which has found common usage throughout the years in both law and custom, still finds wide use in present statutes. By derivation it means not in accordance with the law, born out of wedlock. It is applied to all situations in which birth due to extra-marital relationships results, including those where the mother is unmarried, widowed or divorced, or where her husband could not possibly be the father of the child. (Getz & Kelley, 1956, p. 346)

Writing almost half a century after Frampton and Gall (1955a) had discerned an historical connection between special education and the prevailing social views on morality, Osgood (2000) again highlighted this relationship. Within his history of the Boston schools, Osgood observed that the municipal leaders had used special education to redress a wide range of problems within their community. For this reason, the school administrators had designed special education to accommodate students with multiple types of behaviors. At the beginning of the twentieth century, the superintendent of the Boston Public Schools had made remarks that had seemed to corroborate Osgood's views. That superintendent had recognized that contemporary special educators had been working with students for whom "the cause of the apparent feeble-mindedness is beyond [their] power to discover or remove" (Superintendent Edwin Seaver, 1900, as quoted by Osgood, 2000, p. 3). For this reason, the administrator had instructed the teachers under his authority that potential special learners were to "be reported to the Superintendent of Public Schools, who will call in the expert services of the teachers of the special classes, and, if he deems it best, authorize the removal of the child to one of the special classes" (Superintendent Edwin Seaver, 1900, as quoted by Osgood, 2000, p. 3). On the basis of his research, Osgood had concluded that "Boston emphasized the role of its school system in cleaning up urban blight and assuring the proper education of loyal, productive citizens" (p. 20). Osgood thought that Boston's use of the schools had been particularly significant because it comprised a model through which to address the "problems in urban development [that] were repeated time and again throughout the United States as cities grew and immigration increased" (p. 20).

Teaching Morality to Special Learners

Numerous nineteenth-century educators believed that treatments for disabled persons should be entwined with morality. At the beginning of the nineteenth century, Samuel Tuke (1815a), who was a British scholar, wrote a letter in which he complimented American special educators for recognizing "the importance of moral treatment in the cure of insanity" (p. 9). To further implement this treatment, Tuke encouraged the Americans and his own countrymen to ensure that newly constructed asylums contained chapels. Tuke gave philosophical and practical reasons for following his advice.

> I have known one-sixth of the whole number of patients [at a particular asylum], present at their place of worship in the city, accompanied by their attendants. A still larger number, however, would derive satisfaction from such a practice, who cannot be prudently allowed to quit the bounds of the Institution [*sic*]. A majority

of the patients [at this asylum] are frequently collected together, whilst the super-intendent reads to them. Several attend who are disposed to various irregular actions, and the restraint which such impose upon themselves, is a species of moral discipline, perhaps more highly to be estimated in a curative point of view, than all the famed medicaments of ancient or modern times. (pp. 41–42)

Most nineteenth-century American educators continued to exhibit the religious convictions that had made such positive impressions on Samuel Tuke. Howe (1852), who was an American educator, was convinced that morality was an essential ingre-dient of therapy. In the middle of the nineteenth century, Howe had argued that spe-cial education was worthwhile because it had the potential "of improving the bodily health, of reducing gross animal appetites into human moderation, of breaking up vicious and debasing practices, and of exchanging filthy habits for cleanly ones" (pp. 4–5). He assured his audience that special education would result in "intellect dawning from a night of darkness, and of moral affections springing up from a chaos of selfish desires" (p. 4). Howe highlighted a New Testament passage that he believed demonstrated Christ's commitment to special education.

[Jesus] told us . . . that if one sheep be lost we should leave the ninety and nine and seek until we find it. And shall we not, especially since we need not leave the ninety and nine in the wilderness of ignorance, shall we not seek out lost lambs and gather them into the fold of humanity, that none may be lost, and that we may give account to Him who surely will demand of us his own, and with usury too. [*sic*] (p. 15)

Writing just several years after Howe, Brockett (1855) agreed that immorality was associated with disabilities. In fact, he believed that immorality had been the primary cause of disabilities. Brockett reasoned that "the vast amount of idiocy, in our world, is the direct result of violation of the physical and moral laws which gov-ern our being . . . and . . . the parent, for the sake of a momentary gratification of his depraved appetite, inflicts upon his hapless offspring a life of utter vacuity" (p. 600). Brockett proclaimed that this causative relationship was evident when "the sins of the fathers [were] . . . visited upon their children."

Duncan (1866) was a British scholar who agreed with the Americans' practice of making religion an essential component of special education. Duncan recom-mended that children with disabilities "be taught about religion in its greatest sim-plicity, and also to behave morally in the fullest sense of the word" (p. 154). Duncan even described model programs for achieving these goals.

In the asylum the routine of daily prayer and singing is constant, and the Sunday has its two special services, that is to say, a short sermon or address by the person who has the confidence of the pupils; its divisions should be simple with interesting illustrations, and it should be recapitulated on an after occasion. A service for half an hour in the morning, and another for nearly an hour in the evening, will suffice. . . . The child should be taught to pray to God as his Father in Heaven, to ask pardon of sin, and that the Holy Spirit may make it good and happy. (pp. 167–168)

Duncan reasoned that children with disabilities "are singularly open to temptation and to the influence of evil example, and with them, as with other and more fortunately organized children, practical Christianity is the greatest blessing" (p. 169).

Some nineteenth-century American scholars did not attempt to conceal the direct way in which their Christian beliefs had influenced their attitudes toward special education. For example, Richards (1884) wrote that the work of educating children with disabilities "requires faith,—faith [*sic*] in God as your heavenly Father, and in these little ones as truly the children of God" (p. 419). Richards continued that "with this love and this faith you can conquer any case that I have ever seen." Writing during that same year, Greene (1884) was as forthright as Richards had been when he explained the link between religion and special education.

If civilization is the material expression of the beautiful tenets of Christianity, if the acme of its perfection is reached when society shall believe and practice the code of the Great Teacher. . . . no mere matter of the helplessness, the repulsiveness, or the unprofitableness [*sic*] of these subjects will affect its decision. (Greene, 1884, p. 264)

Walter Fernald (1893) was particularly concerned that persons with disabilities repeatedly would demonstrate negative behaviors. Fernald assured his readers that "the modern scientific study of the deficient and delinquent classes as a whole has demonstrated that a large proportion of our criminal, inebriates, and prostitutes are really congenital imbeciles" (p. 211). Fernald thought that instruction about morality would reduce inappropriate behaviors by the members of these classes. He wrote that such instruction was needed because "the brighter class of the feeble-minded, with their [*sic*] weak will power [*sic*] and deficient judgment are easily influenced for evil" (p. 211). Fernald discouraged "mere intellectual training" and argued for "cultivation of the whole being, physically, mentally, and morally" (p. 215). He added confidently that "the end and aim of all our teaching and training is to make the child helpful to himself and useful to others" (p. 215).

Henderson (1901) was a professor of social sciences at the University of Chicago. In a work that he published originally in 1893, he agreed that morality, religion, and special education were connected. However, Henderson went several steps further than most of his contemporaries. He argued that religion was important to all academic fields in which the scholars were concerned about persons with disabilities. On the basis of this conviction, he directed academic scholars to synthesize religious information with academic information. Henderson then instructed lawmakers and government officials to consult with this new breed of academic scholars, who would counsel them about the best ways to resolve the social problems that disabled persons had created. Henderson thought that the lawmakers and government officials also should consult with university professors about ethical issues, such as the limits of their authority on matters involving disabled persons. Despite his great confidence in university professors, Henderson conceded that the academicians, by themselves, could not solve all of the problems. For this reason, Henderson recommended that lawmakers and government officials seek the counsel of religious leaders, who would help them discover the "real convictions in respect to God and the relations of men to each other as children of a Common Father" (p. 9).

Dealing Firmly With the Morally Disabled

Those scholars who saw a connection between morality and disability did not always agree that religious instruction was the best intervention. For example, Brown (1889) questioned whether students who made exemplary progress in their special education classes should be considered trustworthy. Brown was particularly concerned that even model students eventually would revert to their former behaviors. Believing that disabled persons remained "weak in will" and "weak in moral power," Brown recommended that they be institutionalized for life. Brown thought that draconian measures were necessary to ensure that persons with disabilities were "delivered from temptation" (p. 87).

Risley (1905) also was concerned about the moral recidivism of persons with disabilities. He endorsed sexual sterilization to prevent immoral individuals from giving birth to children with disabilities. Risley singled out "individuals who are the victims of alcoholism" or who had "the opium or cocaine habit" as examples of the immoral individuals that he had in mind. Risley thought that drastic interventions were needed because "the law of heredity is well nigh immutable in its operation" and "the child of the feeble-minded parent is more firmly fixed under the law of degeneracy than were his parents" (p. 94). Risley warned that "the child of the feeble-minded parents or of the criminal and the inebriate begins his vicious life not only earlier but pursues it with a momentum not equaled by the parent" (p. 94). Although many persons thought that institutionalization was an adequate solution for this problem, Risley disagreed with them. He was worried because "it is well known that the parents of these wards are prone to remove them from custody for the purpose of reaping the benefit accruing to the family from their labor" (p. 97). In view of this situation, Risley recommended sexual sterilization, which "at least would render them innocuous" (p. 97).

Rogers (1907), who was a Minnesota physician, was particularly upset by the acts that "moral imbeciles" might commit. Rogers did not list the acts that he had in mind. However, he did attempt to define "moral imbeciles." He defined them as individuals to whom "nothing appeals . . . permanently except that which satisfied their selfish desires" (p. 20). Because he judged these persons to be pathologically selfish and immoral, Rogers recommended "placing them under permanent custody by an act of the court" (p. 20). Even after they had been institutionalized, "moral imbeciles" were to be restricted "from learning to read and write or obtain any form of education that will enable them to increase the amount of mischief of which they are capable" (p. 20).

Sherman (1908), who was a Kentucky school superintendent, wrote an article that he entitled "What the Regular Class Teacher Should Know of Mental and Moral Deficiency." Sherman advised teachers that he had deliberately inserted two types of disabilities into the title of his article because "when one begins an investigation of either, he is very likely to end up with the other" (p. 943). Sherman added that he had "often been surprised" by the fact that both types of disabilities revealed a common set of characteristics and the need for the identical types of treatment. Although Sherman did not specify those common treatments or the manner in which they were to be determined, most of his readers must have assumed that he was condoning the use of harsh interventions.

A year later, Foster (1909), who was a New York judge, wrote an article for a popular magazine in which he made an impassioned case for sexually sterilizing persons with disabilities. Foster admitted that it was "difficult to ascertain the state of public opinion" about this issue because "the question is deemed a delicate one" (p. 572). Fuming at this hypocritical posturing, Foster pointed out that "the details of salacious divorce cases occupy full [newspaper] columns" (p. 572). Foster was equally incensed because some of the opponents of involuntary sterilization had depicted it as a cruel and unusual punishment. With regard to the charges of cruelty, Foster retorted that he could supply "a mass of testimony of physicians 'skilled in the art,' which certainly seems to annihilate this objection" (p. 572). In addition to considering involuntary sterilization cruel, opponents of this treatment had alleged that it was so unusual that it violated rights that were protected by the United States Constitution. Foster countered that the State of New York, which did "prohibit the association of the sexes during their limited period of imprisonment and segregation," did, in effect, "forbid to those convicted of crime the right to propagate their kind" (p. 572). Foster judged that this state precedent was sufficient to dismiss allegations that sterilization was an unusual or unconstitutional measure.

Special Concerns About Immoral Women

Although twentieth-century legislators were worried that disabilities were responsible for the immoral behaviors that many women exhibited, their concerns were hardly novel. Nineteenth-century government officials in Europe and the United States had shared this suspicion. The following passage about the mental problems of young women exhibited this enduring concern. The passage, which was part of a nineteenth-century report, had been reprinted in the *American Journal of Insanity* (Connolly, 1846). The original report had been written by a British scholar.

> Not being called upon for much intellectual exertion, [young women's] great deficiency is for a long time scarcely suspected. They have capacity enough to become skilful in needlework; they go through the routine of school lessons creditably, and sometimes show some skill in drawing, and become accomplished mechanical musicians. But when they arrive at an age in which the affections are expected to be active, and the judgment capable of exercise, they manifest an indifference to their relatives, or an indolence, or apathy, or evident want of power to think and act for themselves. They pursue their occupations in an irregular and desultory manner, neglect exercise, acquire odd, nervous habits, become negligent in dress and behavior, are capricious and irritable, and are found to require constant superintendence. (Unidentified British Scholar, n.d., as quoted by Connolly, 1846, p. 141)

Although the British scholar who had written the preceding passage had employed extremely circumspect language, his intentions must have been apparent to his readers. Those intentions were revealed when this scholar warned that the irregularities about which he was concerned could cause "the undue license of the propensities . . . or the irregular exercise of the affections" (Unidentified British Scholar, n.d., as quoted by Connolly, 1846, p. 145). The author of this passage added that "the resulting eccentricities are humiliating or disgraceful."

Churchill (1851a; 1851b) also had worried about the connection of immorality to disability. He hypothesized that experiences peculiar to females might produce disabilities. For example, he claimed that pregnancy and childbirth could cause "mental disorders" among mothers. Churchill added that women were especially susceptible to disabilities because they "possess a more delicate organization, more refined sensibilities, more exquisite perceptions, and are, moreover, the subjects of repeated constitutional changes and developments of a magnitude and importance unknown to the other sex" (1851a, p. 260).

Seguin was another nineteenth-century scholar who had detected a connection between pregnancy and disabilities. However, Seguin shifted attention to the ways in which abnormal pregnancies could produce disabilities among children.

> [Women's] education—a jumble of that which has made all the male inutilities we have known—has not taught them an iota of womanhood. Their hygiene and habits have disqualified them for motherly functions. City and house narrownesses [*sic*] do not offer more room for a new-comer than their slender pelvises; their tastes run toward niceties [*sic*] incompatible with married life; fecunditation [*sic*] is the result of maladroitness [*sic*]; its product unwelcome, ill-fed, ill-treated, before or disappears in a storm of some sort. (Edward Seguin, 1870, as quoted by Williams, 1909, pp. 190–191)

Seguin had lived in France before he had moved to the United States. On the basis of his early observations, he had concluded that French females who lacked a sense of "womanhood" had mothered many of that nation's disabled children. Furthermore, Seguin was convinced that those French women with immoral lifestyles had conceived the greatest number of disabled children.

Ireland (1877) was an influential European scholar who agreed that the immoral behaviors of adults produced children with disabilities. As such, he recommended that instruction about morality become an essential ingredient of special education. Ireland elaborated that "without moral training mere education of the intellect would only render imbeciles more mischievous and cunning" (p. 322). Although he promised that he would not write "a long vague chapter" about morality and education, Ireland did offer several cautions about the instruction of adolescent females.

> When puberty comes on it creates with those idiots whom it affects a difference between them and ordinary children. Great care and great good sense is required to tide them successfully over the first years, which are the most difficult. Imbecile girls are not safe as a general rule, either in the indigent and crowded quarters of large towns or in large villages, unless they be incessantly watched, which indeed is very difficult. (1877, p. 323)

Ireland had written the preceding passage in 1877. In a subsequent work, Ireland (1898) recapitulated some of the British laws and judicial decisions that pertained to persons with disabilities. He noted that the rape of a girl or young woman would lead to prosecution in the British courts. In contrast, the rape of a disabled adult woman was not considered a criminal offense. To ensure that his readers understood the difference between these two types of incidents, Ireland explained that "the protection accorded to female children is not extended to adult female idiots, for there is a probability of consent, and indeed a possibility of solicitation which cannot be admitted in little girls" (p. 393).

Many citizens worried that disabled persons were inherently immoral. On the basis of this assumption, they believed that disabled persons were prone to parenting children with disabilities. They compounded their faulty logic by assuming that persons who behaved immorally were disabled. They multiplied their errors even further when they concluded that state citizens should imprison the maximum number of immoral persons that their institutions could accommodate. New Yorkers led the citizens of other states in their zeal to incarcerate immoral citizens. They even built new facilities especially for immoral females. In 1885, the New York legislature organized "the first institution in the United Sates established solely for the care of feeble-minded young women during the child-bearing age" (Hart, 1910, p. 4). To help readers understand the rationale for this institution, an observer explained that this specialized asylum was created to save "young women from vice and to prevent the multiplication of defectives" (Hart, 1910, p. 4).

Warner (1894) was a professor who was particularly concerned about "persons convicted of habitual offences against chastity" (p. 291). Before his appointment as a professor, Warner had been the Superintendent of Charities for the District of Columbia and the General Agent for the Charity Organization Society of Baltimore. Warner, who was extremely interested in immoral women, provided precise suggestions about how to deal with them. He recommended that "in case cure or reform . . . should prove to be impossible, they could then be detained during the remainder of their natural lives, working for their own support in a colony" (p. 291). Warner approved of the special women's asylum that New Yorkers had constructed. Realizing that some of his readers might oppose the permanent institutionalization of promiscuous women, Warner attempted to ease their anxieties. He listed several justifications for this type of confinement. For example, he assured the readers that "short commitments for this class of offences are manifestly . . . futile" (p. 291). Furthermore, all wanton females should be treated as if they had mental disabilities because promiscuous women were "especially subject to disorders analogous to feeble-mindedness." Finally, permanent institutionalization would help solve another perennial problem, namely immoral women's peculiar needs for "hospital treatment and prolonged detention" (p. 291).

Talbot (1898), who was a professor of dentistry at Northwestern University, worried about the connection between disabilities and immorality. Talbot concentrated his attention on prostitutes, whom he thought engaged in their immoral behaviors because of "ancestry, habits, [and] perverse instincts" (p. 322). Talbot proclaimed that "prostitutes cannot be cured or reformed by the enforcement of municipal ordinances" (p. 322). He added that, although "those of criminal and congenital type can be taken from their surroundings and placed where they can earn an honest livelihood," they would "soon go back, voluntarily, to their old mode of life" (p. 322). To help his readers understand "the direct hereditary history of prostitutes," Talbot recapitulated portions of the storyline from a novel by Alexandre Dumas.

> [Marie's] paternal grandmother, who was half prostitute, half beggar, gave birth to a son by a country priest. This son was a country Don Juan, a peddler by trade. The maternal great-grandmother was a nymphomaniac, whose son married a woman of loose morals, by whom a daughter was born. This daughter married a peddler, and their child was Marie. She had the confidence-operator tendencies of many of her class. (p. 322)

Obviously, Talbot felt that this fictional narrative resembled the real-world events with which his readers were familiar.

Even the most ardent advocates of expanded institutionalization recognized that this plan had practical difficulties. Lincoln (1903) demonstrated this type of ambivalence. He showed enthusiasm for institutionalization when he stated that "if we had a law for the custodial care of the adult feeble-minded women, a chief danger would be removed" (p. 90). However, Lincoln also demonstrated a sense of political realism when he predicted that few of the immoral women in his own state of Massachusetts would be committed. He explained that "there is not room at present in the state institution for the large number which even Boston could contribute" (p. 90). In view of the dim prospects for institutionalizing all of the women that he wished to see committed, Lincoln devised a backup plan. He resolved that "the next best thing" would be to increase "the moral tone of children" (p. 90).

During the early part of the twentieth century, scholars continued to display censorious attitudes toward females. Lincoln (1903) clearly had demonstrated attitudes comparable to those that most nineteenth-century authorities had exhibited. Writing seven years later, Bullard (1910) did not mask his hostile sentiments. Bullard warned that women with disabilities were "much more dangerous" than the "ordinary male criminal" (p. 15). Bullard explained that these women "become the prey of the lower class of vile men and are the most fertile source for the spread of all forms of venereal disease" (p. 15). Bullard cautioned that women with disabilities were spreading syphilis, which he thought was "on the whole much worse than small pox" (p. 15).

Weidensall (1914) was extremely critical of the female inmates at a New York prison. Sure that these prisoners exhibited cognitive disabilities, he reported that "the mental characteristic most peculiar to the criminal woman . . . is an inexplicable narrowness of her scope of interest" (p. 373). Although he acceded that "what they know may be in quality entirely mature," Weidensall insisted that the female prisoners still had genuine disabilities. To support this assessment, Weidensall pointed out that "in quantity [the women prisoners' knowledge] is almost certain . . . to be but a fragment of the mental content of a normal person of average intelligence" (p. 373).

Instead of focusing her attention on imprisoned adults, Otis (1913) had studied the younger inmates at the New Jersey State Home for Girls. After administering intelligence tests to the 17-year-old females at this institution, Otis noted that many of them had earned scores that she would have expected from 10-year-old children. Although she did not prescribe a specific treatment, Otis did recommend that society protect the female inmates "from the temptations to which they are subject when they go out into the world" (p. 128).

Renz (1914) also studied young females. She examined 100 inmates who were incarcerated at the Girls' Reformatory of Ohio. These inmates, who ranged from 9 to 17 year in age, had been confined primarily for "incorrigibility, disorderly conduct, larceny, street walking, [and] immorality" (p. 37). The editor who had published this report suggested that the girls in Renz's study were those who had been "sent to reformatories because they have gone wrong, and yet whom [*sic*] a closer study shows are delinquent because of mental incapacity" (passage from a prefatory note, editor of the *Training School Bulletin*, in Renz, 1914, p. 37). The editor added that "before going further with the work of our jails, and reformatories and almshouses, our Juvenile Courts and our Charity Organization Societies, we should examine the people with whom we are dealing" (editor of the *Training School Bulletin*, in Renz, 1914, p. 37). Agreeing with her editor, Renz did not suggest corrective actions. However, she did recommend that the prisoners' detention should be extended while additional data were being gathered. Renz explained that "we are not justified in extending to them the privileges and freedom of the normal members of society" (p. 39).

Like several of her professional colleagues, Pyle (1914) wished to learn more about younger incarcerated females. Therefore, she examined 240 inmates at the Missouri State Industrial Home for Girls. These females, who ranged from 7 to 21 years of age, had been incarcerated because they "had been convicted of being vagrants or of some offense not punishable with death or imprisonment for life" (p. 143).

The group included persons who had been "immoral or criminal, or bad and vicious, or . . . incorrigible to such an extent that they could not be controlled by parents or guardians" (p. 143). After she had administered intelligence tests, Pyle concluded that "the standing of delinquent girls is only 65 per cent of that of normal girls" (p. 144). Pyle was convinced that special educators could help these girls. At the same time, she recognized that a proposal to send special educators into reformatories would be extremely controversial. Instead of presenting a detailed plan of intervention, Pyle made an idealistic suggestion. She recommended that any future proposals for solving this problem should "be removed from the realm of politics and brought within the realm of science" (p. 148).

Most of the researchers who had studied immoral women detected a link between disability and prostitution. For example, Goddard (1914), who was a respected behavioral scientist, alleged that "many competent judges estimate that 50% of prostitutes are feeble-minded" (p. 15). Terman (1912), who was a professor at Stanford University, was another preeminent researcher during this era. Terman alluded to evidence indicating that one quarter of all criminals had disabilities. He added that an even greater proportion of "white slaves" had disabilities. Several years after making the preceding observations, Terman (1916) published a report in which he stated that "not all criminals are feeble-minded, but all feeble-minded are at least potential criminals" (Terman, 1916, p. 11). Attempting to validate his earlier estimate about the immorality of females, he opined that it "would hardly be disputed by any one" that "every feeble-minded woman is a potential prostitute" (p. 11). Still later, Terman (1917) alluded to more data to substantiate his sentiments. He wrote that "extensive and careful investigations in large numbers and in divers [*sic*] parts of the United States have furnished indisputable evidence" of the connection between disability and multiple social problems, including "prostitution and venereal diseases" (p. 161).

Doll (1919) agreed with those scholars who saw a link between disability and immoral behavior. He assured his readers that "at least a quarter of criminals and juvenile delinquents are known to be feeble-minded" (p. 190). Doll added that "a very high percentage of professionally immoral women are feeble-minded" (p. 190). Worried that some readers might minimize the significance of these statistics, he lectured them that "mental defectiveness" was the "the most serious single factor in illegitimacy" (p. 190).

Mertz (1919), who was an army psychologist, was sympathetic to Doll's views. He sided with those public officials who had singled out prostitution as "a menace to public health." Mertz added that "the war with its mobilizing of great numbers of men in certain communities has brought to the fore . . . the problem of the prostitute and her control" (p. 1597). Trained as a scientist, Mertz believed the causes of prostitution had to be carefully isolated before a solution could be found. Therefore, he commenced an ambitious research study. Mertz gathered data about the prostitutes who had been arrested near the military base at which he was stationed. He diligently reported that "very few of them were *professional* prostitutes" (emphasis in the original text, p. 1597). He explained that "of the white women, 62 per cent. [*sic*] were married, many of them to soldiers" (p. 1597). Although he may have been convinced that disability was connected to immoral behavior, Mertz interpreted his data dispassionately. For example, he observed that most of the women had received "schooling to the fourth grade" (p. 1599). His objectivity again was apparent when he characterized the typical delinquent woman as only "slightly mentally deficient" (p. 1599).

Draper (1919) was an assistant surgeon in the U.S. Public Health Service. Like Mertz, he was struck by the danger to servicemen from women "who were found conducting themselves in an immoral manner" (p. 642). Draper pointed out that "those found to be infected with venereal disease" had been "committed to the detention hospital for treatment until such time as they were considered noninfectious" (p. 642). However, this precaution turned out to be of little value because the prostitutes were "returned to the police court for trial on the charge for which they were arrested, and invariably released by the judge without further detention" (p. 642). Without formally assessing the prostitutes, Draper concluded that "the vast majority of the whites were of an extremely low grade of intelligence" (p. 643). On the basis of observations and assumptions, Draper urged that "in cases where the mentality is so low as to preclude the possibility of a life other than one of prostitution, it would be an economy and a humanitarian act to commit such individuals to institutional care for life" (p. 643). He believed that severe sentences were justified because the prostitutes were "a far greater menace to the happiness and welfare of society than many murderers who are serving life sentences in our prisons" (p. 645).

Restricting Morally Disabled Women

Scholars, educators, medical personnel, and government leaders all recommended ways to prevent women with disabilities from behaving immorally. Some of them used genealogical patterns to justify the imposition of harsh measures. For example, Kerlin (1877) was a Pennsylvania physician who articulated a callous but popular solution for the problems that immoral women were creating. Kerlin had reasoned that "idiocy and imbecility are dependent *generally* on heredity or prenatal causes; *occasionally* on the diseases or accidents of infancy; [and] *rarely* . . . upon certain debilitating influences" (emphasis in the original text, p. 20). Convinced that the causes of disabilities were usually genetic, Kerlin concluded that persons with disabilities would be "better and more successfully treated in well-organized institutions than is possible at their homes" (p. 21).

Davenport (1911) believed that some critics had worried excessively about disabled citizens' rights to privacy. He explicitly challenged the notion that "feeble-mindedness is a personal private matter" (p. 11). After depicting disability as an instance of inherited disease, Davenport explained why the community had an obligation to take protective measures.

> There is reason for believing that [feeble-mindedness] is one of the oldest traits of mankind—a heritage from his ape-like ancestry. The feeble-mindedness of to-day [*sic*] is (for the most part) the dower of a germ plasm [*sic*] common to hundreds of thousands of kin living and past; and if not controlled, that germ plasm [*sic*] may pass into hundreds of thousands of descendants. How can the product of a germ plasm [*sic*] with such a history regard his traits as purely and private? In a large sense, his germ plasm [*sic*] is a matter of national concern—its source and its possible fate are matters of public interest and concern. (p. 11)

Despite his confrontational stance on this matter, Davenport did recognize the legitimacy of the right to protect the disabled "patient and his family from the distress and burden that empty-headed scandal mongers know how to inflict" (p. 11).

Lapage (1911), who was a British scholar, was as explicit as Davenport when he warned about the genetic basis for disabilities. In the preface to a volume about special education, Lapage explained that his concern about the genetic transmission of disabilities had been one of his primary reasons for writing the book. Selecting language that was remarkably similar to that which Davenport had used, Lapage wrote that "feeblemindedness is an inherited taint handed on from generation to generation, and that every feebleminded person, who is a free and unrestrained agent, may, by becoming a parent, transmit that taint and so affect tens or hundreds in future generations" (p. vii).

Wallin (1914) was an American educator who developed a set of questions to help teachers distinguish those students who required special education. The questions that Wallin selected demonstrated his sensitivity to the prevalent views about genetics and disabilities. Parents or caregivers were to be asked about "defects, conditions or diseases found in the child's brothers, sisters, mother, father, maternal and paternal great-grandparents, grandparents, aunts, uncles, first and second cousins" (p. 446). The inherited "defects, conditions or diseases" for which teachers were to search included nervousness, epilepsy and "mental queerness." The inherited traits also included immorality, which was revealed by criminal acts, alcoholism, or promiscuous sexual behaviors.

Figure 1.4 is a genealogical chart from an early twentieth-century textbook (Woodrow, 1923). This illustration depicted an individual's progeny from two women. One of these women was "normal" while the other was "feeble-minded." The male's sexual relationships with the "normal" woman had produced 500 descendents, all of whom were normal. His sexual relationships with the disabled woman had resulted in another 500 descendents, who were predominantly abnormal. The genetic implications of these data were evident. However, readers were sure to notice the chart's additional information, such as that referring to the morality of the father and his progeny. The chart revealed that the male never actually married his "feeble-minded" companion. The chart also revealed that this relationship produced two female grandchildren who were "sexually immoral."

Murchison (1926), a professor of psychology at Clark University, recommended that criminals be given severe sentences. He maintained that "no moral or legal principle would be violated if the third penitentiary conviction carried an automatic death penalty" (p. 291). To convey the basis for his recommendation, Murchison explained that "if it is moral to hang a murderer, it is even more moral to hang the habitual robber or burglar" (p. 291). He insisted that severe sentences be imposed on all criminals, irrespective of the degree of intelligence that they demonstrated. As such, Murchison endorsed "uniform punishment for the insane, the feeble-minded, and the young" (p. 291).

Walker (1930) was concerned about the "delinquency of defective girls." He stipulated that "sexual offense characterizes the delinquency of our defective group, which means that, from the point of view of public health, eugenics, and social standards,

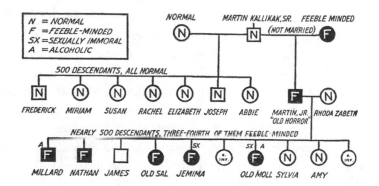

Figure 1.4. Genealogical Chart from an Early Twentieth-Century Textbook.

the defective delinquent offers a more serious problem than does the average delinquent girl" (p. 202). Walker proposed two interventions for this problem. One of these was sterilization. Aware that many persons considered this procedure to be inhumane, Walker offered humanitarian and economic rejoinders.

> For many high-grade defectives, not promiscuous in their habits, sterilization and parole seem much more humane and eliminate unnecessary expense. Many of these, if sterilized and protected in a home or even if married, could settle down to a peaceful and happy routine. (pp. 206–207)

In addition to sterilization of young women with disabilities, Walker (1930) espoused incarceration. He wrote that "for the promiscuous, segregation is essential" (p. 206). Walker supported this remedy so strongly that he advised judges to "commit [young women] on a basis of mental defect without waiting for further serious delinquency" (p. 207). Anticipating a public backlash against those judges who followed his advice, Walker recommended that the judges for the juvenile courts should "be appointed rather than elected" (p. 207).

Bridgman (1930) reviewed eight studies that had been conducted from 1913 to 1915 and that had linked moral delinquency with disability. Some of the researchers in these studies had concluded that the majority of persons who were being arrested for prostitution had disabilities. Agreeing with these researchers, Bridgman was convinced that decisive governmental intervention was required. He recommended that school personnel identify children who were "incapable of developing normally" and then "make adequate plans for them before they become delinquent" (p. 54). Bridgman hoped that those delinquents "who need special care or supervision can be provided for permanently" (p. 54).

Baker (1927) also had been concerned about the sexual promiscuity of disabled persons. He had warned his readers that "no great civilization, without the foundation stone of good mental health, can long survive" (p. 178). Baker therefore suggested that "we render true and noble service to our brother man" (p. 178). Those readers who believed that the preceding statement revealed egalitarian sentiments misunderstood Baker's use of the term "brother man." Baker had been referring only to those "brother men" who did not have disabilities. In fact, Baker applauded the first American sterilization law, which had been passed in 1907. He also paid tribute to the 23 states that had enacted comparable laws during the subsequent two decades. Baker boasted that "any state in the union can now make a eugenical [*sic*] sterilization law which the courts will hold constitutionally sound" (p. 175).

Arnold (1938) presented data about the 1000 patients who had been "eugenically sterilized" at a Virginia asylum. This group had comprised 609 females and

391 males. Seven hundred and eighty-one of these patients had been committed because they were feebleminded. Arnold wished to give his readers and understanding of the perspective from which he had examined these cases. He was convinced that "heredity and environment both play an important part in the production of feeble-minded persons" and that "when both heredity and environment are bad, there is only a very remote possibility that the child born in those circumstance will develop into a normal adult" (p. 63). Because he was certain that involuntary surgeries could reduce inappropriate behaviors that were heredity-based, Arnold searched the patients' records for evidence that their disabilities had been part of multigenerational patterns. After he had completed his examination, Arnold was disappointed because "the histories in several hundred of these cases were not nearly so [*sic*] complete as we would desire" (p. 60). Even though he failed to locate relevant evidence, Arnold concluded that the surgeries had been appropriate. Somewhat unconvincingly, he rationalized that "in spite of [poor records], we *know* that 50 percent of these one thousand patients had a definitely bad family history" (emphasis in the original text, p. 60). In an article that he published a year later, Arnold (1939) asserted that he had found "no reason" to change his earlier conclusion. In fact, he had come to realize that "economy" provided an additional justification for the sterilizations. Arnold explained that the sterilizations were economical because they enabled the staff at the Virginia asylum "to place in their own or foster homes some 632 of 1,000 patients upon whom we had operated, thus relieving the State of Virginia of the burden of their care and support" (1939, p. 173).

Not all state officials sterilized institutionalized patients. In fact, some of them had to deal with legal mechanisms through which the citizens of some states could exit asylums. The state officials in Maryland provided an example. Kanner (1938) summarized information about those persons who had left the Maryland State Training School for the Feebleminded. The persons in question had been released from 1911 to 1933 in response to writs of *habeas corpus*. Kanner recognized that "the writ of habeas corpus is one of the major guarantees of individual freedom" and that it was "rooted in the Magna Cara and provides redress for any person detained against his will in a prison, institution, hospital or any other place"(p. 1013). In spite the storied history of this legal safeguard, Kanner protested its "unwise application" by judges who "need enlightenment in matters of psychiatric and communal importance" (p. 1031). To underscore his point, Kanner recounted details about the 102 inmates whom judges had released from the Maryland State Training School for the Feebleminded.

Thirteen [of the inmates who were released] made a satisfactory adjustment; 11 died; 17 were remanded, and 5 released again after being returned to the school;

17 acquired tuberculosis, syphilis or gonorrhea; 8 were committed to mental hospitals; 29 became prostitutes; 6 served prison terms of more than 3 months duration; 51 married; 165 children were produced, of whom 33 were illegitimate, 18 died, 30 were placed in orphanages and foster homes and 108 are incontestably feebleminded. (p. 1030)

Kanner (1938) believed that his data demonstrated that miserable lives awaited those inmates who were released from asylums. He thought his data also showed that wretched lives awaited the children that the released inmates would parent. Jones (1936), who had reviewed an earlier version of Kanner's research report, praised it for focusing the public's attention on a serious problem. Jones wrote that Kanner's study had generated more publicity "than the feebleminded problem has had in the newspapers in Baltimore City in the whole history of that city's existence" (p. 1031). As for the conclusion that Kanner had drawn from his research, Jones labeled it a "statement of incontrovertible fact" (p. 1032).

Disabled Delinquent Youths

Scholars, educators, medical personnel, lawmakers, and members of the public fretted about the threats from persons with disabilities. They were concerned that promiscuous females would seduce righteous and moral males. They worried that both disabled females and disabled males would parent handicapped children. They feared that the disabled females and the disabled males would engage frequently in a full range of immoral and criminal acts. They became even more anxious after some behavioral theorists predicted that an epidemic of inherited diseases was festering.

Although some individuals were extremely disconcerted by gloomy eugenic theories, the opponents of these theories dismissed the predictions. In fact, the opponents believed that changes in the environments of delinquent youths could transform them into wholesome members of society. Like those individuals who subscribed to genetic determination, the opponents of this theory wanted to identify delinquents early. Both groups supported early identification and early intervention for the same reason: they wished to reduce the mischief in which delinquent youths otherwise would engage. However, both groups lacked the critical data that they needed to argue their cases convincingly. For example, they could not confirm the number of persons that their respective treatments would affect. They could not furnish this figure because Europeans and Americans had been unable to make a controversy-free count of youths with disabilities.

Near the end of the nineteenth century, Daniel Tuke (1878), a British scholar, had attempted to calculate the number of persons with mental disabilities. He had judged that this matter was of "profound interest" because it was related to a broader question, namely "whether among the peoples of the highly civilized portions of the globe at the present day, more persons do or do not become insane than among the nations of antiquity" (p. 1). Tuke proposed to answer this question by making an historical analysis of the "acknowledged" causes of mental disabilities, the degree to which these factors had been "in full force in the ancient world," and the degree to which these factors currently were prevalent.

More than a decade after he had completed his 1878 investigation, Daniel Tuke (1894) still wished to compute the current number of persons with mental disabilities. However, he decided to make the calculation differently. On the second occasion, Daniel Tuke looked at the number of British asylums that had been operating from 1870–1890. He also examined the number of persons who had been admitted to the asylums during this period. After analyzing these data, Tuke detected increases in the number of asylums and in the number of persons that they were accommodating. Tuke speculated that the increases might have resulted from improved diagnostic techniques, more effective treatments for persons with disabilities, and the longer life spans of patients. However, he eventually dismissed all of these explanations. He wrote that that, as "potent as these causes may once have been, they have now lost their force" (p. 2). As an alternative explanation, Tuke suggested that "a lower type of mental disease has developed in recent years" (p. 2). This recently emerged strain of disability had made such an impression on the staffs at asylums that they had changed their admission criteria. To validate this opinion, Tuke procured supportive testimonials from long-serving asylum superintendents.

Wilmarth (1898), who was the Superintendent of the Wisconsin Home for the Feeble-Minded, was another scholar who wanted to investigate the number of persons with mental disabilities. He decided to expand the scope of Tuke's British survey and then extend it to the United States. Wilmarth was interested in the number of individuals with disabilities who had been placed in asylums or several other types of institutions. Wilmarth then consulted the 1880 and 1890 national censuses. These censuses respectively revealed that 76,000 and 96,000 feebleminded Americans had been detained in asylums, hospitals for the insane, prisons, reformatories, poor houses, or schools. After gathering this information, Wilmarth conceded that it was inconclusive. For example, he suspected that patients with "higher grades of imbecility" had been "often not recognized" (p. 1277). Other problems resulted from the idiosyncratic, poorly documented, or completely undefined procedures through which students had been admitted to the school-based programs.

These same drawbacks extended to the procedures that had been used to admit persons to the other types of facilities, including the asylums.

Many professionals had detected procedural shortcomings similar to those that Wilmarth had observed. At the beginning of the twentieth century, Davenport (1911) had proposed to circumvent these problems through an extraordinary census. The census that he had in mind would count only feebleminded individuals. Davenport admitted that this initiative, even were it to be implemented, might fail. He explained that "a complete and accurate census of all feeble-minded persons is at present impracticable" because of faulty "methods of detecting feeble-mindedness" (p. 9). The problem of accurately detecting disabilities was compounded by the disagreements among professionals about basic terms such as *feeblemindedness*. Davenport suggested that the extraordinary census he was championing should focus on those persons who had been admitted to specialized schools or asylums, which were the institutions where the supervisory personnel had "true insight" about which inmates were feebleminded. Without explaining how additional data could be gathered accurately, Davenport suggested "the inclusion in statistics of the feeble-minded of those who are cared for in county poorhouses" (p. 9).

Like many earlier professionals, Pollock and Furbush (1917) saw the need to accurately count the number of persons with disabilities. Although they already had access to data about the persons with disabilities who were being kept in "almshouses," Pollock and Furbush questioned the validity of this information. They also questioned the validity of data about patients who were confined in jails and reformatories. Because of their reservations, Pollock and Furbush decided to limit their research to the patients in state and private asylums. They reported that these institutions had admitted patients under four general classifications: insanity, epilepsy, chronic inebriation, and feeblemindedness. Although Pollock and Furbush recognized that many of the records they had examined were flawed, they still relied on them. They calculated that 37,200 feebleminded persons were being confined in American asylums. As an indication of just how tenuous their conclusion was, Bernstein (1918) presented a startling statistic just a year later. Bernstein reported that "the very conservative estimates of the State Board of Charities" indicated that New York state alone encompassed 30,000 "feeble-minded and socially unfit individuals" (p. 150).

Restricting Disabled Delinquent Youths

At the beginning of the twentieth century, medical personnel, educators, scholars, lawmakers, and members of the public had different impressions of the danger that disabled youths posed. They also had different ideas about the most effective way to contain that danger. Their attitudes were influenced by the distinct ways in which they viewed the origin of disabilities.

Most people were convinced that delinquent youths were genetically predisposed toward negative behaviors. Although they were not optimistic about eradicating these genetic tendencies, the scholars who subscribed to this explanation believed that instruction about morality might control some aberrant behaviors. In an essay that he published in *Popular Science Monthly*, Taylor (1906) distinguished "difficult" boys from "backward-minded" boys. Even though he believed that these two types of children could be "clearly" differentiated, Taylor discerned "grounds on which they may become merged." For example, "backward" youths could devolve into "difficult" ones if their inclinations toward apathy, laziness, secretiveness, and immorality were not managed carefully. Taylor believed that instruction about morality was an essential component of the management that was needed.

Donkin (1911) was a member of England's Royal Commission on the Care and Control of the Feeble-Minded. Like many other European educators, he assumed that heredity determined delinquent behaviors. He assured readers that legislation was needed to manage the problems created by "the hereditary nature and consequent propagation of mental defect" (p. xviii). If these problems were not managed effectively, Donkin warned that "the certain prospect of large numbers of mentally defective children" would result in misery for the children themselves and "multiform |sic| evil to others" (p. xviii). As far as "effective" interventions were concerned, Donkin and many likeminded colleagues recommended mandatory institutionalization. Some of Donkin's European and American allies, who wished to take an additional measure to restrict persons with disabilities, urged that mandatory sterilization should supplement institutionalization.

A group of educators did believe that environmental factors could be responsible for delinquency. These educators claimed that problem behaviors, which were caused by the environment, could be eliminated by changes in the environment. They hoped that temporary confinements in reform schools might provide the environmental pretexts for those changes. They argued that the reform schools were not only effective but also extremely accessible. Snedden (1907) made this point within his extensive report about American reform schools. Referring to data collected in 1903, he indicated that 96 schools had been responsible for "34,422 inmates, taught by 644 teachers and cared for a force of 2,275 men and women as matrons, guards, teachers of trades, [and] parole officers" (p. 7).

The 75-year-old institution known as the Philadelphia House of Refuge was one of the reform schools that Snedden (1907) had examined. The directors of the Philadelphia House of Refuge believed that the development of religious and moral habits would change the lives of incarcerated youths. The central roles of religion and morality within the Philadelphia House of Refuge were clarified in the remarks that an administrator had made during that school's 1832 opening ceremony.

> The Refuge is not a place of punishment; it is not a provision simply, nor even principally, for the security of society against offence. . . . [It] invites the children of poverty and ignorance whose wandering and misguided steps are leading them to swift destruction, to come to a home where they will be sheltered from temptation, and led into the ways of usefulness and virtue. (Remarks made by John Sergeant, President of the Board of Managers at the Philadelphia House of Refuge, 1832, as quoted by Snedden, 1907, p. 12)

The George Junior Republic in Freeville, New York, was another reformatory at which the staff encouraged delinquent youths to develop wholesome habits. This New York institution had tried "to duplicate in miniature the economic, civic and social life of a real democracy" (Jennings & Hallock, 1913, p. 471). The primary goal of the George Junior Republic had been to "make industrious, self-reliant, moral men and women" out of youths who were "wayward, criminal or immoral" (Jennings & Hallock, 1913, p. 472).

Rather than write about the children in reform schools, Devereux (1909) reported about socially aberrant children in the public schools. She believed that "the great need of those children . . . was to make them less like little animals—to instill humanity into them" (p. 47). Devereux explained that the children she had examined were "freakish in disposition and temperament . . . selfwilled [*sic*], passionate, [and] malicious . . . largely because they have not the sense of their fellows to see when it was expedient to be 'good' " (p. 47). Devereux was convinced that an appropriate regimen of daily instruction, even if it were provided as part of a public-school program, would alter the behaviors of youthful delinquents.

Maennel (1909) was a German educator who had doubted the degree to which genetic factors caused juvenile delinquency. His own professional experiences had convinced him that many "backward children" had been harmed by destructive environments. He explained that delinquent children came from families where "the parents are addicted to strong drink, dislike work, lead immoral lives, or have come into frequent touch with the strong arm of the law" (p. 71). Even though the causes of their behavior may have been environmental, Maennel feared that some of their consequences were irreversible. He provided teachers with several analytical devices for evaluating the backgrounds of their students. One of these instruments, which delved into morality, directed the instructor to look for indications of egoistical, altruistic, ethical, and religious impulses.

Farrell (1908–1909), who had established special education in the schools of New York City, partially shared Maennel's perspective about the causes of delinquency. Unlike Maennel, Farrell admitted that her ideas were "not the result of any theory" (p. 91). Although Farrell developed a program that may have lacked a theoretical base, she did recognize that negative environments could foster "many and serious problems in truancy and discipline" (p. 91). Maennel and Farrell both believed that the manipulation of environmental factors could reduce some of the inappropriate behaviors that youths with disabilities exhibited.

Some scholars maintained that juvenile delinquency resulted primarily from heredity. Others believed that it resulted chiefly from the environment. Rogers (1912) was convinced that both explanations had merit. He recommended that professionals use intelligence tests to detect some of the inherited sources of delinquency. Rogers cautioned that tests might not be able to confirm "borderline cases" of delinquency. Nonetheless, he insisted that the value of tests was "unquestioned in the filed of juvenile delinquency, for quickly detecting the large number [of delinquents] that present . . . low [intellectual] levels" (p. 144).

Like Rogers, Guy Fernald (1912b) believed that both inherited and environmental factors could cause problem behaviors. He also believed that tests could help educators determine whether heredity or environment had caused a particular delinquent's behaviors. He added that the tests also would reveal the type of instruction that educators should prescribe for that patient. With regard to the instruction, Guy Fernald recommended that "high grade defectives" receive "the rational, educational and humane treatment which their condition demands" (p. 534). He recommended a different intervention for the "so-called 'Moral Insane' cases, criminal degenerates and criminal sexual deviates" (p. 526). Guy Fernald thought that these groups should be "committed for segregation" (p. 526). He also recommended institutionalization for "defective unmarried females who have borne one, two, three or even more feeble-minded children" (p. 526). After he had recommended this harsh treatment, Guy Fernald did add a provisional note. He wrote that some immoral women might "be restored to their friends and society after a longer course of custodial and educational care that is required for the reform of the ordinary delinquent" (p. 526).

Like Guy Fernald, MacMurchy (1915) worried about the morality of persons with disabilities. MacMurchy was a Canadian educator who advised her constituents to be on special guard against "moral imbeciles." She defined "moral imbeciles" as "persons who from an early age display some permanent mental defect, coupled with strong vicious or criminal propensities on which punishment has had little or no deterrent effect" (p. 23). MacMurchy agreed with Guy Fernald on another point. She thought that the moral reprobates were "a great danger to the community" (p. 23). In view of this danger, she recommended that they "should always be under permanent care" (p. 23).

Even those persons who showed understanding and tolerance for persons with disabilities were extremely cautious when they were recommending more humane treatments. Walter Fernald (1919), the superintendent of the Massachusetts School for the Feebleminded, exclaimed that "it is now generally understood that the feebleminded and the progeny of the feebleminded constitute one of the great social and economic burdens of our modern civilization" (p. 566). He concluded that "an intelligent democracy cannot consistently ignore a condition involving such a vast number of persons and families and communities, so large an aggregate of suffering and misery, and so great economic cost and waste" (p. 566). In spite of his censorious attitudes, Walter Fernald did not believe that all persons with disabilities were genetically predestined to lead institutionalized lives. He insisted that "the average family chart of the patients admitted . . . is not a 'black' chart" and that "the average defective coming to the institution is not the child of a feeble-minded parent or parents" (Walter Fernald, n.d., as quoted by Wallin 1922b, p. 22). Using this insight to guide him, Walter Fernald joined the coalition that was promoting special education as the way to help disabled learners cultivate appropriate habits.

Berry (1923), who was the Director of Special Education for the Detroit Public Schools, had placed numerous children with disabilities in that city's general educational system. However Berry's remarks about these children were as cautious as those that Guy Fernald had made several years earlier.

> While it may be true that the mentally retarded child is a potential sinner, it is equally true that he is also a potential saint, and whether he becomes a saint or a sinner will depend in large measure upon the type of training he receives in the home and in the school. And in his education the emphasis should be placed primarily upon the acquisition of right habits, and only secondarily upon the acquisition of knowledge. (p. 766)

Although Berry's remarks may have been cautious, they still revealed his fundamental confidence in public-school programs.

Shifting Attitudes Toward Persons With Disabilities

During the nineteenth century, scholars and professionals began to shift their views of persons with disabilities. The public joined this trend. These shifting attitudes influenced the ways in which students with disabilities were treated in the schools. However, once educational changes began to transpire, these changes actually caused society's attitudes to shift even further. As such, changing attitudes simultaneously may have been a cause and an effect of innovative educational programs.

Changing attitudes were apparent within those professional and charitable organizations that sponsored services for students with disabilities. The members of these organizations initially had shared a common set of assumptions. They were certain that many individuals with disabilities represented grave threats to society. They were sure that the sinful behaviors of parents had caused the problems that their disabled children exhibited. They believed that controlling sexual promiscuity would reduce the spread of disabilities. They believed that many individuals with disabilities needed to be permanently assigned to asylums or jails. They believed that children and adults with disabilities required instruction about morality and religion. Although the preceding suppositions never disappeared, less censorious assumptions gradually emerged.

Even during the nineteenth century, less censorious attitudes had begun to appear. Some European scholars attested to these attitudes. John Batty Tuke (1868) noted that "many good authorities" in Scotland were advocating alternative types of facilities for "harmless lunatics and idiots" (p. 916). John Batty Tuke thought that these alternative facilities could accommodate many of the patients that currently were confined in asylums. He indicated that the emerging type of care would be more economical than asylum-based programs. John Batty Tuke added that, "better still, it would ensure partial liberty to very many who are now subjected to the more rigid discipline of the asylum" (p. 918).

Daniel Tuke had contributed significantly to some of the social and educational changes of the late nineteenth century. Daniel Tuke (Bucknill & Tuke, 1858; Tuke, 1872; 1878; 1885) was a professor who had written influential texts about mental disabilities. He (Tuke, 1892a; 1892b) also had edited a comprehensive, two-volume set of reference books: *A Dictionary of Psychological Medicine, Giving the Definition, Etymology and Synonyms of the Terms Used in Medical Psychology, with the Symptoms, Treatment, and Pathology of Insanity and the Law of Lunacy in Great Britain and Ireland*. Otis (1917) had referred respectfully to Daniel Tuke as "the great authority on mental diseases." Although they were writing nearly a century after Otis had offered this encomium, Goldney and Schioldann (2002) agreed that Daniel Tuke continued to occupy "an important place in the history of the medical psychology of the English speaking world" (p. 23).

Despite the praise that colleagues gave him, Daniel Tuke did not always reciprocate. For example, he had not concealed his skepticism about the ways in which most of his peers had been identifying patients with disabilities. In fact, he had remarked irreverently that their shoddy practices had made it safe "to be assumed that the deity is sane but whether anybody else is, is a debatable question" (Daniel Tuke, n.d., as quoted by Otis, 1917, p. 191). Otis (1917) applauded Tuke's derisive comments. He was convinced that the problems of Tuke's era had stemmed from a lack of discipline by researchers and academicians. Otis advised his readers that that these problems still were unresolved.

Alfred Binet was a French psychologist who had devised an immensely popular intelligence test. Binet also had authored a textbook in which he and a colleague had addressed the ways in which professional and social attitudes toward disabled persons were shifting. Assuming a Marxian vantage, they (Binet & Simon, 1914) advised their readers to support progressive social changes.

> [The responsibility to help persons with disabilities] does not rest solely upon a sentiment of humanity. It is dictated equally by our own pressing personal interests; for unless, within a reasonable time, satisfaction is given to the just demands of the nine-tenths of society who are actually working for wages very little in harmony with their efforts and their needs, we already foresee that a violent revolution, from which the "haves" have very little to gain, will shake society to it very foundations. . . . The movement referred to, of which we see only the beginning, but which will result, let us hope, in an amelioration of the lot of the great majority, is now being directed to the education of the mentally defective. (pp. 1–3)

Binet and Simon viewed persons with disabilities from a politically progressive viewpoint. Although they may not have been as politically radical, more and more of their contemporaries adopted progressive viewpoints. This trend continued throughout the twentieth century.

Changing American Attitudes

Shifting attitudes toward persons with disabilities could be detected in Europe before they were discernible in the United States. Nonetheless, some early changes could be detected in the United States. Writing in the United States, Brown (1889) had questioned many of the progressive assumptions of his European colleagues. He specifically challenged those European scholars and educators who believed that persons with disabilities could lead independent lives. Despite this skepticism, Brown did respect those professionals who had established special schools within European asylums. On the basis of the success in Europe, Brown deemed it "an axiomatic proposition that the State should educate all its dependent children"

(p. 86). Brown credited newly established programs in the United States with educating "thousands" of Americans with disabilities between 1848–1889. These statistics convinced Brown that a "goodly number" of persons with disabilities could be educated. Brown added that teachers could further increase the effectiveness of their efforts if they would "individually instruct" students with disabilities.

During the early part of the twentieth century, Groszmann (1906) noted that many American educators had adopted the progressive attitudes of their European colleagues. Groszmann wrote that the Americans had begun "to realize that a very appreciable faction of children exists in our schools to-day [*sic*] whose educational needs are being overlooked under the usual public or private school régime [*sic*]" (p. 425). Although American educators historically had recognized cases of severe disability, Groszmann thought that it was "only within the last five or six years that a fuller recognition of this condition of comparatively minor deviation has been observed" (p. 425).

Many of the American educators who were skeptical about special education believed that a deep, wide, and possibly unbridgeable chasm separated special learners from other students. Gilbert (1906) employed a subtle type of rhetoric to dispute this assumption. He began his argument by dispassionately observing that "no school is composed of normal and evenly developed minds" (p. 45). For precisely this reason, Gilbert questioned whether any school's staff should "take account of all of these irregularities and treat each child independently, basing the course upon his state and his consequent needs" (p. 45). Gilbert discouraged administrators from converting a school into a "pathological institution," a classroom into a "ward," or a desk into an "invalid's cot." He stated emphatically that school administrators should resist the temptations to create specialized clinics. Instead they were to preserve their traditional educational missions and recognize that "common sense is as important in school as elsewhere" (p. 45).

Farrell (1908–1909) was the public-school administrator who had developed the special educational programs for New York City. As one might expect, she exhibited extremely progressive dispositions toward students with disabilities. Convinced that special students were not a discrete group of learners, she advised teachers to avoid instructing them in separate buildings. Instead, the special educators were to insist that their students have access to classrooms that were "part and parcel of the regular school." Although Farrell asserted that "I need not justify this I am sure," she still offered several rationalizations that teachers could use when they were confronting tradition-minded principals and superintendents. For example, the teachers could explain that placing special learners in the academic mainstream would establish "a relation between the ungraded class children and others which is most desirable"

(p. 94). They also could note that mainstream placements provided "encouragement to the parents," who would see that "the work which we are doing in these [special education] classrooms does not differ essentially from that done in other grades of the school" (p. 94). Finally, they could stress that these changes would alter the social dynamics in ways that would reduce the "stigma" associated with special education.

Bolton (1912) wrote with pride about the expanding educational services that were available to children with disabilities. With regard to students who were visually impaired or deaf, he noted that "every state has either established schools for its own or has made provisions for their education in adjoining states" (p. 63). The legislators of New York gone further and established "a statute that any blind student attending a college, university, or technological institution, other than a school for the blind, shall have a reader provided for him at an expense not to exceed $300 per year" (p. 63). Bolton acknowledged that "so general has the education of the blind and deaf become that most people probably believe that nothing more remains to be done in this direction" (p. 63).

Although he applauded the steps that had been taken to help students who were visually impaired or deaf, Bolton (1912) still worried about students with other types of disabilities. He demanded that all special learners, including "juvenile offenders," be treated in an "enlightened" manner. He added that the administrators in several public school systems already had adopted the enlightened viewpoint. After challenging his readers to identify the cities where these administrators resided, Bolton answered the question for them. He singled out New York, Chicago, Boston, Philadelphia, Cleveland, Detroit, Buffalo, Washington, Baltimore, and Seattle as cities where school administrators had established noteworthy programs.

Wright (1915) was the founder of a private school for deaf children. As one might expect, he had progressive views about students with disabilities. He began his book, *What the Mother of a Deaf Child Ought to Know*, with the acknowledgement that the parents of a deaf child should be prepared to demonstrate "patient devotion and courageous effort." Wright categorically stated that "while deafness is a serous misfortune, it is neither a sin, nor a disgrace, to be ashamed of" (p. 1). Wright advised parents that solicitous attention to their children's needs would assure them futures of "comfort and usefulness."

Otis (1917) was distressed by the punitive fashion in which many students with disabilities had been treated. After acknowledging that the states had responsibilities to protect their "citizens from palpable injurious influences," Otis pointed out that they also had the duty to provide "an opportunity for development, a chance to realize that 'freedom, equality and pursuit of happiness' which is declared to be the birthright of us all in this country; hence the public schools and the libraries, and other public educativ [*sic*] measures" (pp. 192–193). After assessing the status of children with physical impairments, Otis concluded that state leaders had done a fairly good job of providing educational opportunities to this group. He thought that legislators had demonstrated an impressive commitment to students with speech, hearing, or vision problems. However, Otis felt that they had done significantly less for "crippled and deformed" children. So that they would understand the goals toward which they should aspire, Otis described the advanced facilities and equipment at a Boston school for children with physical disabilities. He approvingly noted that most of that school's students "are conveyed to the school and returned to their homes daily," that "all receive a substantial dinner at noon," that "adjustable desks and special seats are provided," and that "cots for rest periods and special gymnastic training are given" (pp. 195–196). Otis recommended that every community establish special schools with comparable equipment and services.

Progressive educators who opposed imprisonment and institutionalization recognized that they had a responsibility to suggest alternative treatments. Witmer (1919) suggested that academic learning could be the basis for these new treatments. To demonstrate the reasonableness of this proposal, he published an account of a young boy named Don. The byline that accompanied this publication summarized Witmer's account.

> Don was, in the eyes of his parents, a hopeless boy. At 2 years and 7 months old he could hardly walk; he could speak only 8 words. Everybody thought him feeble-minded, of such low grade as to be beyond hope. Against his own judgment, Professor Witmer (perhaps the ablest child psychologist in the United States) took Don, and in this remarkable article he tells what he did with him. To-day [*sic*] he is absolutely a normal child and presents a case, in scientific annals, second only to that of Helen Keller. (Byline accompanying an article by Witmer, 1919, p. 51)

The preceding passage had introduced a detailed report. In the actual report, Witmer (1919) had used a popular writing style to describe an innovative educational approach. This approach required instructors to introduce, monitor, and modify their academic plans. This complexity of Witmer's approach was revealed in the section of the report that dealt with reading instruction.

> I did not push his reading in the second year as I had done in the first. Attempting to teach him phonic analysis as this is employed in language work, I made up my mind that he was not ready for it. Primarily I was not interested in having him read, write and cipher efficiently. I was interested only in arousing his latent capacity to do this work. I had no desire to produce an unbalanced monster. (Witmer, 1919, p. 123)

Although his philosophy was preeminently child-focused, Witmer selected a some-what insensitive metaphor to explain it. He wrote that "you can coax most children, some of the time at least, by appealing to their interests and desires, even as the hunter entices the deer to come into gunshot by appealing to its curiosity" (p. 51).

The advocates for progressive approaches to special education disagreed with those individuals who had portrayed disabled persons as threats to themselves and their communities. Whereas their opponents cited statistics to demonstrate that disabled individuals were genetically disposed to lives of misery and failure, the advocates for progressive education presented data that revealed very different prospects. The following passage illustrates the type of rhetorical strategy that these advocates employed.

> A study of 350 children from [special education] classes who had been in train-ing in the New York City Schools between 1907 and 1914 and [who] had left the schools . . . shows that 192, over one-half, were succeeding at occupations along the line of that which they had learned in the special class work [*sic*]; and that 86 others were employed and cared for at home helping at industrial occupations which were done in the home along the line of work they had learned to do at the schools, such as sewing, artificial flower-making, etc., 31 had been employed but were at present temporarily out of employment and only 18 had proven to be so defectiv [*sic*] that it was necessary to send them to institutions, and only 3 had fallen into the hands of the law for social offenses. (E. E. Farrell, 1917, as paraphrased by Bernstein, 1917, pp. 209–210)

Wallin (1922b) believed that persons with disabilities should not be treated in punitive fashions. Moreover, he suspected that the backers of punitive treatments had relied on faulty research. For example, Wallin alleged that researchers had misclassi-fied the participating subjects within those studies that had linked disabilities to crime. Wallin feared that these tainted studies had been used to institutionalize or imprison many innocent persons. Wallin then described a project in which researchers had employed sound methodology. These researchers had determined that "the median intelligence level of 3,328 white criminals corresponded exactly with the median intel-ligence of our white soldiers" (Wallin, 1922b, p. 34). Wallin wrote that these data had led him to realize that persons with low mental aptitude were not predisposed to crime. The accuracy of this insight was reinforced when the researchers revealed that African American criminals actually had scored two points higher on intelli-gence tests than African American soldiers.

Like Wallin, Mateer (1924) was concerned that the research linking disability with crime. She attempted to correct the popular perception that the vast major-ity of juvenile delinquents were "feeble-minded or even backward." Although

Mateer conceded that "mental endowment [was] probably an important factor in the evolution of the child who is potentially a law-breaker," she did not think that a child was inherently dangerous because he or she had a disability. To the contrary, Mateer insisted that the child with a disability presented "no traits that are not easily understood and explained" (p. vii). Sure that error-filled research reports had misrepresented the danger of children with disabilities, Mateer wrote that "there is no such thing as a bad child" (p. x). Instead, she suggested that a child who appeared to be bad "does not know any better or else he cannot help it" (p. x). As for the persons who wished to incarcerate children with disabilities, Mateer pointed out that such recommendations were ethically and financially untenable.

Scheidemann (1931) was another scholar who disputed the assumption that persons with limited intelligence would become criminals. To emphasize his point, Scheidemann reviewed data about the intelligence of incarcerated criminals. In an analysis of 21 youths who had been truant from school and then arrested for crimes, she noted that the subjects displayed a median IQ score of 84. The median IQ for the five youths who had been convicted of arson was 74. The two murderers in the group respectively had scored 56 and 68 on IQ tests. Scheidemann concluded that a lack of intelligence had not predestined any of these youths to crime. However, she did believe that their degrees of intelligence had influenced the types of criminal actions in which they had engaged. Scheidemann reasoned that "interest which is based upon intellectual ability determines at what a person will be successful in crime, just as [it does] in occupations and school work" (p. 452).

Changing Attitudes Toward Curriculum

During the twentieth century, more and more educators began to suggest that children with disabilities would benefit from specialized curricula. In contrast, nineteenth-century educators had insisted that information about morality overshadowed academic information. Inskeep (1926) explicitly disagreed with the nineteenth-century assumptions. She argued that "dull and retarded [children] should be taught everything they are capable of learning that will function with life" (p. 1). She added that "for them, as for normal children" the goal of instruction should be the creation of "self-controlled, self-supporting citizens" (p. 1). As to those critics who thought that this new approach was too expensive to be implemented, Inskeep pointed out that ten percent of the students in regular education classrooms annually repeated one grade's instruction. She suggested that the funds that were being "wasted on repeaters" could be used to subsidize special educational programs. Inskeep wrote emotionally that the redirected funds would create changes that were "far better than to leave these children cowed by failure, the prey to every evil suggestion that promised success" (p. 2).

Four years after she had made the preceding observations, Inskeep (1930) restated the same points in a manner that was even more politically provocative.

> The school and the jail are the only places *where forced attendance is legal.* All must attend school because the right kind of education will enable children to adjust them in the best possible manner to life. If they fail *singularly* in this adjustment, they must go to jail. With education compulsory, the attendance is no longer limited to children from educated homes. . . . The one time [*sic*] marplot on the otherwise fair day in the school or the home becomes its most interesting occupant, because he presents to teacher and parent the vital and absorbing task of scientifically adjusting a *human being* so that he will function normally. (Emphasis in the original text, Inskeep, 1930, pp. vii–ix)

Pressey and Pressey (1928) agreed with Inskeep that inappropriate educational practices had harmed learners. They decried those antiquated education procedures that had "developed inferiority complexes which were a handicap and source of unhappiness throughout life, as result of repeated failure in school" (p. 298). Pressey and Pressey adjured teachers to join "the modern movement for adjustment of school work to intelligence" (p. 298). Once the teachers had become members of this philosophically and pedagogically cohesive movement, they could provide "simple work" with which an individual student could be successful and "in which he can take pride."

Descoeudres (1928) was a French educator who had written a book, *The Education of Mentally Defective Children*, which had been translated into English, distributed in the Untied States, and influenced American teachers. In her book, Descoeudres had included a chapter on moral training. Although this was her volume's shortest chapter, she reassured her readers that the brevity of the section was "not because we minimize its importance" (p. 294). This explanation initially might have comforted the proponents of religion-based and morality-based curricula. However, ideological zealots eventually must have recognized that Descoeudres had an extremely broad notion of morality. For example, she discouraged attempts to promote morality through "words or precepts or even stories, however well adapted to the circumstances and mentality of the child" (p. 294). Descoeudres judged that moral training "depends far more upon the *living example of the teacher*" (emphasis in the original text, p. 294). As readers progressed through this book, they leaned that Descoeudres equated morality with a child-centered philosophy. The author's empathetic attitude was underscored when she wrote that "what is needed above all . . . in the training of the backward is a moral personality" that would stir a teacher "to interest himself in the misfortunes of childhood" (p. 294).

Descoeudres had made the preceding remarks in a book that she published in 1928. Her comments obviously revealed her personal attitudes. Additionally, they reflected society's changing attitudes toward the treatment and education of children with disabilities. Traditionally, advancing the interests of children with disabilities had been only one feature of a politically and educationally complex model of social services. Community safety and morality were other features of that model. Those nineteenth-century pioneers who had devised the early approaches to special education had placed a heavy, and sometimes exclusive, emphasis on community safety and student morality. However, the importance of community safety and student morality diminished during the twentieth century. This change in educational priorities was apparent when Frampton and Rowell (1938) wrote the introduction to their special education textbook. After observing that disabilities could be classified as physical, mental, or social, these authors stated that the social category currently included "the largest number of persons and the widest ramification of problems" (p. 2). Frampton and Rowell noted that this category was especially difficult to summarize "due to rapidly shifting points of view" about it.

Summary

Some nineteenth-century educators believed that genetic factors caused disabilities. Others saw immorality as their source. However, the members of both groups agreed that they were in grave danger. They thought that disabled persons should be sent to asylums, prisons, or reformatories. They recommended that they then learn about religion and morality. Reform-minded educators protested that restrictive settings were cruel and inappropriate. They also raised protests about religion-centered instruction. They wanted disabled students to learn academic, vocational, and life skills. They believed that they could master these skills in school-based day-care programs. They defended their approach as a way to promote humane care, economical services, and noninstitutionalized living.

2

Designing Facilities and
Preparing Teachers

Feeble-minded children in public school are a menace to the normal children.

—Doll, 1919

After acknowledging their responsibility to care for persons with disabilities, members of the public had to designate the facilities at which they would provide that care. Many of them preferred asylums. However, the living conditions at the asylums were deplorable. Additionally, their high costs made them impractical. Political moderates searched for alternatives that were less oppressive and less expensive. They experimentally sent some adult patients to communal residences. As for disabled children, the political moderates began to send them to the public schools. They then devised innovative techniques to train the staffs for the new facilities.

Searching for Facilities

Most nineteenth-century European citizens assumed that persons with disabilities were menaces. On the basis of this assumption, they wished to send them to asylums, prisons, or reformatories. Humanitarian citizens challenged these plans. Confident that disabled persons were not as dangerous as they had been depicted, the humanitarians attempted to care for them in new ways. For example, they began to send patients to less restrictive facilities such as private schools, church-based centers, clinics, hospitals, and group homes.

DeFelice (1851) described an experimental facility that a physician had established in rural Switzerland. DeFelice, who had visited this facility in the middle of
the nineteenth century, recounted the experience in a letter to the *New York Observer*.

> The buildings are well arranged; there is a large eating-room [*sic*], a well ventilated
> school-room [*sic*], a farm attached to the establishment, &c [*sic*]. Nothing is
> expended upon luxuries; but all for convenience and comfort [*sic*]. (DeFelice,
> 1851, p. 239)

Guggenbuhl, who had designed the Swiss facility and its curriculum, had emphasized vocational training. However, he had believed that religious instruction should
be intertwined with the vocational training. Guggenbuhl supposedly had formed this
conviction after meeting a disabled person who was repeating the words of a prayer.
DeFelice (1851), who had interviewed Guggenbuhl, alleged that this chance meeting had evoked sentiments that "decided the whole course of the doctor's life." The
religious implications of Guggenbuhl's sentiments were apparent in the remarks that
he had made immediately after this incident.

> Are not these beings our brethren? Have they not an immortal soul like us? And
> since they have some idea of God, do they not deserve our sympathy and atten-
> tion? If these Cretins should be from their infancy the object of regular and suit-
> able treatment, if religion, charity, science, were employed to restore them from
> their abasement, is it not probable that some at least might be rescued from their
> wretched state? (Dr. Guggenbuhl, n.d., as quoted by DeFelice, 1851, p. 238)

DeFelice (1851) noted that the curriculum at Guggenbuhl's institution had been
designed to help students prepare for vocations. At the same time, he recognized that
it had been designed to teach students about "the idea of God,—of [*sic*] salvation by
Jesus Christ,—of [*sic*] pardon offered us in the gospel,—of [*sic*] eternity" and "all the
great doctrines of Revelation [*sic*]" (p. 241). Convinced that Guggenbuhl had correctly
analyzed and responded to his patients' most pressing needs, DeFelice asked rhetori-
cally, "What do they need more?"

Greenwell (1869) was a British Scholar who had written one of the early
books about special education. Like Guggenbuhl, she did not conceal that Christian
principles were the foundation for her professional dispositions. She stressed these
principles in examples throughout her monograph. On the first page, she citedthe
Biblical psalm, "He shall be favorable to the simple and needy" (p. 1). On the book's
title page, Greenwell quoted a passage in which a Christian scholar had explained
the spiritual rationale for charitable actions.

To help where no one helps, to try to effect improvement where no one attempts it: to espouse the cause of Humanity [*sic*] wherever it lies imprisoned, languishing in body or spirit, in things of earthly or of eternal life, this is Christianity.— Wherever [*sic*] these good deeds flourish, Christ will find them and gather them into his bosom. (Herder, n.d., as quoted by Greenwell, 1869, title page)

Daniel Tuke was a widely respected British scholar with a reputation for making insightful observations about persons with disabilities. However, his observations frequently were as acerbic as they were insightful. In the preface to his history of special education, Daniel Tuke may have startled readers when he advised them that his book should be purchased by those "who may reasonably suspect that they have the seeds of madness sown in their own constitution" (1878, p. vii). Although many of his contemporaries had detected ways in which religion had nurtured positive attitudes toward disabled persons, the irascible Tuke (1882) challenged their contentions. In fact, Tuke used the term "medico-ecclesiastical" to categorize institutions at which persons with disabilities had been treated deplorably by religious zealots. He explained that the care at the "medico-ecclesiastical" facilities was "a curious compound of pharmacy, superstition and castigation" (Tuke, 1882, p. 1). Tuke added that "demoniacal possession was fully believed to be the frequent cause of insanity" and that "exorcism was practiced by the Church as a recognized ordinance" (p. 1).

Americans Search for Facilities

Like the Europeans, nineteenth-century Americans had assigned persons with disabilities to several types of facilities. Initially, they had placed them in prisons, reformatories, and poor houses. As asylums and specialized hospitals became available, they sent them to these sites. At the very end of the nineteenth century, they began to assign them to the public schools.

Writing during the second quarter of the nineteenth century, Mann, Taft, and Calhoun (1832) had commented on the facilities to which handicapped persons in Massachusetts were being sent. They noted that officials in Massachusetts had been imprisoning those persons who were judged to be "dangerous to the peace or safety of the good people" (p. 17). Once they had been imprisoned, disabled patients were treated poorly. To emphasize this point, Mann, Taft, and Calhoun quoted some of the remarks that had been made by a visitor who had observed incarcerated patients.

[One imprisoned person with a disability] had a wreath of rags round [*sic*] his body, [*sic*] and another round [*sic*] his neck. This was all his clothing. He had no bed, chair or bench. Two or three rough plank [*sic*] were strewed around the room; a heap of filthy straw, like the nest of swine, was in the corner. He had built a bird's nest of mud in the iron grate of his den. Connected with his wretched apartment was a dark dungeon, having no orifice for the admission of light, heat or air, except the iron door, about two and a half feet square, opening into it from the prison. (Passage from a report to the Secretary of the Massachusetts Commonwealth, 1929, as quoted by Mann, Taft, & Calhoun, 1832, p. 20)

Not all disabled Massachusetts citizens were imprisoned. Mann, Taft, and Calhoun (1832) reported that the state officials had taken "no special cognizance" of those handicapped persons who were not "furiously mad" and who had the ability to pay for private care. Mann, Taft, and Calhoun had underscored the ways in which wealth and social status influenced the treatment of disabled patients. The relevance of these two factors was equally apparent in the ways that "town pauper lunatics" were treated.

[Town pauper lunatics] are mostly confined in poor-houses, by order of the municipal authorities, though it has been the practice of some towns to make private contracts with the keepers of jails and houses of correction, to take their insane poor at a low price, and imprison them in some of their unoccupied cells, where no person has been held responsible for their treatment, nor has the law designated authority to any one to examine into their condition. Other towns have annually offered the keeping of their insane poor at auction, and struck them off to the lowest bidder, by whom they have been taken and treated with various degrees of attention or of cruelty, according to the character of the individual, who, in this competition for the profits of keeping them, would be likely to prevail. (Mann, Taft, & Calhoun, 1832, pp. 16–17)

A decade after Mann, Taft, and Calhoun (1832) had made their critical comments about the treatment of persons with disabilities, several positive social developments could be detected. For example, government officials had built asylums in some of the states that previously had none. Even in those states that still lacked asylums, the officials at least had begun to discuss whether they should build them. The American architects who were hired to work on these projects had opportunities to consult with experienced European professionals Ray (1846), who had been the superintendent of asylums in Maine and Rhode Island, took advantage of these opportunities. He met with European architects who had designed the facilities in England, France, and Germany. Ray employed a highly editorialized style of writing when he was reporting about the progress that he had observed in Europe. This style was evident when he wrote about the bedrooms in British asylums.

> The sleeping-room of the pauper patients, are a trifle smaller than ours, with high unplastered walls, and a small window. . . . To us they have a naked, cheerless, prison-like aspect, but we must bear in mind that to most of those who occupy them, they are far more comfortable than any they have been accustomed to, and therefore convey a very different impression to their minds. It would be a misplaced kindness to furnish poor patients with accommodations very much better than they ever knew before, and to which their own poverty-stricken abode, when they return to it, would present a painful contrast. (pp. 319–320)

Brigham (1845) was an expert on the design of specialized facilities. After he was contacted by the New Jersey officials who were about to erect an asylum, he discouraged them from meeting with European builders. He assured them that North America had enough architectural talent to guide their new project. Brigham advised them to pay special attention to an asylum that had recently been erected in Rhode Island. He also instructed them to examine some of the newer Canadian facilities. In both the Rhode Island and Canadian cases, Brigham detected the influence of medical superintendents. He wrote that the architects had consulted these superintendents about "the internal arrangement of the building" (p. 285). Brigham urged the New Jersey authorities to assure that their medical staff had a significant role in the design of their new asylum. If this adjuration were ignored, he predicted that "many small but important particulars will be omitted, and which will have to be added afterwards at great expense" (p. 285).

Brigham's admonitions about construction had been straightforward and reasonable. More than 30 years after Brigham had made his remarks, Seguin (1878) also provided advice about the design of facilities. However, Seguin's advice was significantly more abstract than that of Brigham. It also was more controversial. Seguin was concerned that the structure of buildings could influence the ways that the supervisors and caretakers treated their patients. He wrote philosophically that "if ideas create architecture, architecture reacts upon its mother-idea, to develop, distort, [and] even kill" that mother-idea. To substantiate this contention, Seguin relied on his own observations about the influence that the architecture "of the insane asylum has exercised on the theory and practice of the treatment of insanity" (p. 60). Seguin singled out a particularly progressive asylum in New York as a prototype for other institutions. He wrote that the New York asylum had been built "without prenotions [*sic*] contracting beforehand its ideals" (p. 60).

Religious Convictions Influence American Facilities

Brigham (1845; 1847; 1848) was a scholar who had recommended solicitous, patient-centered, humane care. However, he was aware that his contemporaries had different opinions on this matter. In fact, he anticipated that some of them would reject his suggestions. Brigham (1847) predicted that religious zealots would prefer punitive treatments. To establish a basis for this prediction, he reviewed the ways in which persons with disabilities had been harmed by religious zealots in the past. He reported that persons with disabilities "were condemned to death or to imprisonment for life as heretics, some were hung for practicing witchcraft, and vast numbers were burned as sorcerers, or for being in league with the devil" (p. 3). Brigham thought that these outrageous practices had "for the most part passed away." Nonetheless, he could identify some nineteenth-century scholars and educators with religious attitudes that were so peculiar that they continued to enkindle distrust of disabled persons.

In the middle of the nineteenth century, Howe (1852) had been extremely suspicious of persons with disabilities. Howe's attitudes seemed to have been linked to his religious convictions. After noting an increasing incidence of disabilities among citizens in Massachusetts, Howe had objected that "surely it cannot be in the Divine design that there should *always* be one idiotic person to every thousand of whole mind, any more than that there should always be so many blind, so many dumb, so many insane, [or] so many cripples" (emphasis in the original text, p. 6). As an alternative to divine intent, Howe suggested that "every one of these cases arose from disobedience to His Laws." On the basis of the preceding logic, Howe recommended a "return to obedience" as the best way to reduce the frequency and the "wretchedness" of disabilities.

Writing near the end of the nineteenth century, Talbot (1898) urged members of the public to treat disabled persons humanely. As an initial step, they could assign disabled persons to clean and comfortable facilities. Talbot was especially concerned that his advice would be opposed by individuals with pernicious religious attitudes. He alleged that "the religious sense marked by assigning malign occult powers to natural objects and forces" had "exposed weakly or deformed offspring, charged to evil powers, to death" (p. 2). Talbot then gave a current example of the inappropriate attitudes that he had in mind. He noted that "against degenerate children charms are still used by the 'witch-doctors' among the 'Pennsylvania Dutch' " (p. 2). Talbot denigrated the Pennsylvania Dutch as "on the level of culture of the early seventeenth century [*sic*] middle class, if not a little below it" (p. 2). However, he did acknowledge that the attitudes of the Pennsylvania Dutch were not typical of most nineteenth-century citizens.

Like Talbot, Polglase (1901) urged the public to support humane treatments at comfortable facilities. Polglase also agreed with Talbot that persons with disabilities historically had been victimized by religion. In fact, he concluded that many of them had been executed because they were depicted as "possessed of devils." Polglase quipped bitterly that these hapless victims may have been executed in order to ensure that they would receive immediate as well as "eternal punishment" (p. 186).

Although some Christians did oppose the movement to treat persons with disabilities more humanely, many individuals who were devout Christians joined the movement. For example, Brigham (1847) had excoriated those religious zealots who wished to treat disabled persons harshly. At the same time, Brigham did not suppress his own Christian beliefs. He recommended that persons with disabilities receive "respectful and kind treatment under all circumstances" (p. 1). Brigham thought that "in most cases" they would benefit from "manual labor, attendance on religious worship on Sunday, the establishment of regular habits and of self control," and the "diversion of the mind from morbid thoughts" (p. 1). A year after he had made the preceding statements, Brigham (1848) called attention to "the deplorable and neglected condition of the Idiotic [*sic*] and Imbecile [*sic*], and the urgent necessity of establishing Asylums [*sic*] and Schools [*sic*] for their comfort and improvement" (p. 19). Brigham referred to the model of care that he was espousing as "benevolent exertion." Aware that some persons would disagree with him about the value of his approach, he assured them that they eventually would applaud its "useful and pleasing results."

In the middle of the nineteenth century, Brace (1857) had been searching for facilities at which persons with disabilities would be treated with kindness and dignity. He also hoped that these facilities would be relatively inexpensive. Finally, he hoped that they would be currently available. He thought that the American vocational schools might meet all of these conditions. He pointed out that many vocational schools had been built. Furthermore, more were being constructed. Brace was impressed that some of the staffs at these schools already had begun to admit students with disabilities. After he had listed practical reasons for school administrators to admit disabled students to vocational facilities, Brace identified an equally important spiritual incentive.

> Will not, in the far-away dim Eternity, a day come in which a voice, sweeter than all earthly music, shall sound to the depth of your soul, bringing rich peace and joy, and saying, "Inasmuch as ye did it unto one of the least of these, ye did it unto me!" Ye did in unknowing, unseen, for one of the poorest and basest of your fellows, and ye find in that day, it was done for humanity, for Christ, for God. (p. 19)

Two years after he had made the preceding remarks, Brace (1859) gave his support to another innovative type of care. He endorsed the practice of removing juvenile delinquents from the cities and requiring them to work for "good families in the country." Brace again used religious tenets to justify his plan. He wrote that it was worthwhile because "the family is God's Reformatory; and every child of bad habits who can secure a place in a Christian home, is in the best possible place for his improvement" (p. 12).

Scholars Influence American Facilities

Some nineteenth-century citizens approved of the asylums, prisons, and other restrictive facilities in which many persons with disabilities were confined. Their approbation was connected to their belief that this type of confinement protected society. Other nineteenth-century citizens opposed restrictive facilities as cruel and inhumane. A third group comprised individuals who philosophically opposed restrictive facilities but who pragmatically endorsed them. The persons in the third group reluctantly justified restrictive facilities as expedients that were needed to prevent disabled persons from harming others and themselves. The social, religious, and political attitudes of the era influenced the dispositions of the persons in all three groups. The opinions and arguments that scholars advanced also influenced their dispositions.

Peterson (1896) was one of the many scholars who expressed his opinion about persons with disabilities. Peterson's basic opinion was simple: disabled persons were extremely dangerous. It is impossible to determine the extent to which Peterson's opinion influenced the public's attitudes. It also is impossible to detect the extent to which prevailing public attitudes persuaded Peterson to adopt his opinion. Irrespective of its origin, Peterson's opinion was extremely popular at the end of the nineteenth century. In a paper that he read at a meeting of the American Medico-Psychological Association, Peterson highlighted the damage that disabled children and adults inflicted. The inevitability of this damage was a key feature of his argument.

> DESTRUCTIVENESS, a propensity even in normal children at an early age, is an especial attribute of all classes of idiots. In those of low degree it is automatic . . . but in some individuals of the superior grades there seems, at times, to be a vicious satisfaction in inflicting damage or injury, which may even lead to the manifestation of homicidal proclivities or a tendency to arson. (p. 13)

Gegenheimer (1948), who was a social worker at an asylum, looked back on the early years of special education. She estimated that assumptions such as that which Peterson (1896) had articulated did have a significant influence on the public's attitudes. Furthermore, Gegenheimer believed that these nineteenth-century assumptions continued to have an impact for decades. Gegenheimer gave specific examples of the assumptions to which she was referring.

> Authorities and laymen took it for granted that feeble-minded persons must have lifelong segregation. It was believed that most of them were of hereditary type, often of low social levels, that they should be kept from propagating large families, many were criminalistic [*sic*] and that the majority were a burden to society. (p. 93)

Writing during the second decade of the twentieth century, Goddard (1914) assumed that all of his readers would agree with him about the desirability of segregating persons with disabilities. Goddard reasoned that segregation was needed to prevent disabled individuals from harming their neighbors. However, Goddard extended this argument by proposing that even community nuisances be institutionalized. Goddard described the individuals that he had in mind.

> Every community has its quota of people, who, because of their failure to act in harmony with those who are definitely working for the welfare of society, may perhaps be designated as undesirable citizens or ne'er-do wells; while not paupers, they often have to receive assistance from others; while not criminal, prostitute or drunkard, are still shiftless, incompetent, unsatisfactory and undesirable members of the community. (p. 18)

Goddard concluded his remarks about community nuisances with a truism that he hoped would be persuasive. He stated that "a goodly proportion of these ne'er-do-wells" should be institutionalized because they were "of such relatively low mental level that they cannot adapt themselves to their environment as the majority do [*sic*]" (p. 18).

Attitudes Toward Crime and Disability

Many groups listened carefully to those behavioral scientists who had investigated the connection between disability and crime. Law enforcement personnel, judges, and wardens were particularly interested in their advice. Many of the behavioral scientists had made recommendations about treatments that would reduce the number of crimes that disabled persons committed. For example, many of them recommended the lifetime commitment of any disabled persons who had committed crimes. However, some of them went further. Believing that all persons with disabilities were preordained to commit criminal acts, they recommended that even the disabled persons who were law-abiding should be sequestered.

In a review of the research about disability and crime, Clarke (1915) focused his attention on just that portion of the professional literature in which researchers had connected disability to prostitution. Clarke concluded that this connection was "sufficiently striking to demand more careful mental examination of preadolescents and more elaborate provisions for the discovery, training, and protection of children whose minds are not normally developed" (p. 364). Terman (1916), who was a preeminent psychologist of this era, reported that "one of the most important facts brought to light by the use of intelligence tests is the frequent association of delinquency and mental deficiency" (p. 7). Although he did not use this "important fact" to make specific political recommendations, Terman assured readers that the systematic use of intelligence testing could "result in curtailing the reproduction of feeble-mindedness and in the elimination of an enormous amount of crime, pauperism, and industrial inefficiency" (p. 7). In the byline to another article about the interrelationships among crime, disability, and testing, an editor had referred to the ongoing professional arguments about these topics. This individual wrote that disputants had either sanctioned or contested the increasing use of psychological tests "as tools for the criminological laboratory in the courts" (Kohs, 1915–1916, p. 860).

Wallin (1917) was one of the many scholars who had examined the research literature on disability and crime. He noted that "during the last few years it has been repeatedly affirmed that 'every feebleminded child is a potential criminal' and that 'the majority of criminals are mentally defective' " (p. 585). Sympathetic to these generalizations, Wallin alluded to studies demonstrating that "from 50 per cent to 85 per cent and even 90 per cent of different groups of delinquents and criminals have actually proved upon examination to be feebleminded" (p. 585).

During the first two decades of the twentieth century, the debates over crime and disability became more strident. Additionally, the number of participants who were involved in the debates increased. For example, Crafts (1916–1917) provided 210 citations of scholars who had conducted research about the relationship of crime and feeblemindedness. Shortly afterward, Bevis (1918) conducted a similar review. Summarizing the conclusions from the numerous studies on this topic, Bevis noted that feebleminded individuals "lack self-control . . . yield easily to temptation . . . usually fail to earn an independent living . . . drift easily into immorality and crime . . . transmit their defects from parent to child . . . [and] have an unusually high birth rate among them in the absence of proper moral guidance" (pp. 322–323). In view of these conclusions, Bevis thought that feebleminded persons "need proper institutional care" (p. 323). Writing several years later about "moral imbeciles," Shuttleworth and Potts (1922) opined that a child with this type of disability was the "despair of his parents, the *bête noire* of the institution, the perplexing puzzle of the jurist" and "the ill-fated product of inherited nervous instability and ancestral criminal instincts" (p. 241). In his book on intelligence and crime, Murchison (1926) explained that he would forego the trouble of developing a detailed bibliography of the books and reports that had connected crime and disability. However, Murchison only restrained himself because so "many excellent bibliographies" were "already accessible" (p. 8).

Attitudes Toward Crime and Disability Influence Facilities

When they were forming opinions about persons with disabilities, politicians and members of the general public were influenced by several assumptions. One of these assumptions posited a connection between disability and crime. In addition to affecting their general attitudes, this assumption influenced their deliberations about the facilities to which disabled persons should be assigned. Draper (1919) was a case in point. Draper had been concerned not only about the connection of disabilities to crime but also about its connection to venereal disease. He believed that both crime and venereal disease could be reduced by placing immoral women with disabilities in "detention hospitals." Even though he staunchly supported these facilities, Draper admitted that "the cost of the detention hospital is the most serious obstacle in the path of its development" (p. 645). For this reason, he recommended that the federal government provide the money to build new detention facilities. Two years after Draper had made these observations, Cornell (1921) conducted a survey to determine the total number of asylums, special hospitals, and other restrictive facilities that state governments were supporting. After he was able to document only 41 institutions, Cornell attributed this paucity to the high costs of construction and operation.

Doll (1919) had reported that "the prevalent method of relieving the communities of the burden imposed by feeble-mindedness is to place mental defectives in institutions for permanent custodial care" (p. 191). However, Doll pointed out that all of the current custodial institutions were filled to capacity. The ensuing shortage of facilities had prevented the further implementation of this plan. For this reason alone, Doll recommended less expensive alternatives. These alternative facilities would include group homes in which "the adult life of the mental defective is controlled at the cost of supervision only" (p. 191).

As for the many children with disabilities, they could be placed in public schools. The schools were plentiful, affordable, and accessible. The schools also were sites that the parents of disabled children found attractive. Most parents did not want their children separated from them. They opposed programs that required their children to reside at distant asylums or hospitals; they preferred programs that would offer daycare in the children's own neighborhoods.

Although public-school facilities were affordable and popular, Doll had reservations about them. He warned that "feeble minded children in public school are a menace to the normal children" (p. 191). Even if they addressed the physical dangers, school-based special education programs might create other types of hazards for the students without disabilities. Doll believed that one of these hazards was "the neglect of the normal children" that resulted from "the extra attention which must be given to the defectives" (p. 191). Another danger was the "undesirable consequences" that the "normal" students demonstrated after they had interacted with their disabled peers.

Economic Considerations Influence Facilities

Many nineteenth-century citizens thought that the cost of caring for persons with disabilities had become excessive. Samuel Tuke (1815a), who had pioneered innovative models of care in Great Britain, had addressed this issue forthrightly. He discouraged the in-home care of persons with disabilities because this could expose the family members "to great personal dangers." He endorsed asylum-based care as the only appropriate alternative. In spite of his strong convictions about the merits of asylums, Samuel Tuke realized that private asylums were extremely expensive. Therefore, he advised any administrators who wished to build new asylums to ensure that their facilities were government-funded. He thought that this subsidy was essential because "the expense and difficulty of private management . . . may bring to ruin a respectable family" (p. 5).

Although he believed that asylums provided the best type of care for persons with disabilities, Samuel Tuke (1815a) recognized that the current number of asylums could not accommodate all of the individuals whom society judged to be dangerous. This problem was compounded because the incidence of disabilities appeared to be increasing. It also was compounded by the fact that many newly classified patients seemed to be nuisances to society rather than threats to it. The possibility of permanently incarcerating all dangerous persons and all nuisances was out of the question.

John Batty Tuke (1868), who was the superintendent of an asylum, reported that "great anxiety is already felt in many of the districts of Scotland at the gradually increasing number of pauper lunatics" (p. 916). Although the Scottish citizens to whom John Batty Tuke had referred were reluctant to allow disabled persons to remain at large in the community, they showed even "greater reluctance" to the payment of the higher taxes that were required to institutionalize more disabled persons. As such, John Batty Tuke wished to find a less expensive alternative to asylum-based care. He thought that communal residences could solve this problem. Referring to the communal living programs as "cottage treatments," he pointed out that they were not only effective but preeminently affordable.

John Batty Tuke (1868) had described the publicity that had surrounded the Scottish debates about the increasing number of persons with disabilities, the danger that these persons represented, and the cost of caring for them. A decade later, another member of the Tuke family corroborated the political attention that persons with disabilities were receiving. Daniel Tuke (1878), a British scholar, wrote about the interest of the "public at large" in "questions relative to insanity." He indicated that this interest had grown into "a remarkable feature of the present day" (p. vii).

Economic Considerations Influence American Facilities

European citizens worried about the increasing number of individuals with disabilities, the danger that they posed, and the cost of caring for them. When they attempted to solve these problems, they considered a full range of political considerations. Nonetheless, they often relied on financial considerations when they had to designate the type of care and supervision that individuals with disabilities should receive.

Like the Europeans, the Americans worried about persons with disabilities. Like the Europeans, they considered political factors when they had to propose solutions. Like the Europeans, they frequently deferred to financial factors when they designated the ways in which patients should be treated. Warner (1894), who was an American professor of economics, wrote straightforwardly about the interplay of finances and care.

> Farmers or others are paid to care for . . . idiots, epileptics, incurables, incompetents, the aged, abandoned children, foundlings, women for confinement, and a considerable number of the insane, the blind, and the deaf and dumb. . . . In some populous cities the almshouses are hardly more than enlarged specimens of this same type. (pp. 141–142)

Perceptions about costs influenced the ways in which the general public treated persons with disabilities. They also influenced the types of facilities to which it assigned persons with disabilities. Recognizing the importance of this factor, advocates and opponents of special education raised financial issues when they addressed the public. The advocates of special education pointed out that school-based care was less expensive than institution-based care. Although the opponents of special education did not question this assertion, they did question whether those reduced costs were in proportion to the benefits. Believing that disabled children behaved aberrantly because of inherited traits, they predicted that those children who were exposed to school-based treatments would not be cured. Consequently, they would remain liabilities to their communities. Although the proponents of institutionalization recognized that institutionalization was much more expensive than special education, they depicted it as the only genuinely effective intervention. In fact, some of them wished to raise the cost of institutionalization by pairing it with mandatory sexual sterilization.

Wilmarth (1898), the Superintendent of the Wisconsin Home for the Feeble-Minded, had written about the perils of hereditarily transmitted mental defects. He was convinced that these dangers justified the institutionalization of individuals with disabilities. Nonetheless, Wilmarth warned that even an institutionalized person "may go home to his family during his better periods form a hospital and resume his family relations and cause the birth of other beings who stand much more than a chance of a miserable life" (p. 1278). In addition to questioning the effectiveness of institutionalization, Wilmarth judged that its cost constituted a great "burden" to society. Wilmarth used a metaphor to illustrate an effective and financially reasonable solution for this problem. He alluded to the farmer who can "exterminate the weeds most thoroughly from the ground, which should bear only life-supporting grain, by seeing that they do not seed" (p. 1278). To be sure that his readers had not missed his point, Wilmarth added that "the surgeon may yet be called upon to follow the example of the farmer, and by operating, guard society from the contamination and burden of the increasing number of those whose lives should never be begun, and by a comparatively safe operation make parentage impossible" (p. 1278).

Like Wilmarth, Alexander Johnson (1899) was preoccupied with the threats that persons with disabilities posed. Like Wilmarth, he supported asylums, hospitals, and restrictive facilities. Johnson wrote that restrictive "institutions can take . . . undesirable and hurtful citizens and make of them, or of many of them, self-supporting members of a separate community, and at the same time avert the dangers of reproduction" (p. 471). Despite his endorsement of restrictive facilities, Johnson admitted that "the cost of these schools has been great in the past, and when we consider the number to be provided for—at least ten times as many as are now in the institutions—the total cost would appear prohibitory" (p. 471). This financial problem was likely to increase because of "the belief of the proprietors of some small private institutions . . . that, to achieve good results, the number [of students] in any one school should be very small" (p. 466). The consequence of this ideal-istic belief, which some persons wished to extend to public institutions, was a man-agement policy that had "a ratio of cost so high that only remarkable results in the improvement of the pupils could justify its being defrayed from public funds" (p. 466). A third factor that had raised expenses was the reluctance of some admin-istrators to release their patients once they had "reached the age limit of the insti-tutions." Johnson explained that "in every institution there began to be an accumulation of inmates at or past the legal age limit, who yet were so manifestly unfit for self-control that the managers felt it a wrong both to them and to the com-munity to dismiss them" (p. 466).

Johnson (1899) had indicated that he supported asylums, specialized hospi-tals, and the other types of restrictive facilities. At the same time, he had conceded that the costs were high. Whereas Wilmarth (1898) had suggested that involun-tary sexual sterilization could be an effective, affordable, and expedient alternative to institutionalization, Johnson hoped to find a more humane option. Johnson sin-gled out the establishment of special educational programs in American public schools as a potential solution for this problem. Johnson expressed his hope that these new scholastic programs would demonstrate that "the improvables [*sic*] can be cared for, with decency and humanity, at a very moderate ratio of expense, by utilizing the labor of the trained higher grades" (p. 471).

Religion, scholarly convictions, and finances were some of the issues that had influenced the nineteenth-century deliberations about the types of facilities to which persons with disabilities should be assigned. These same elements continued to influence political dialogues during the twentieth century. However, the cost of financing care assumed greater importance as the number of persons requiring care increased. To reduce the expense of asylum-based care, persons with disabilities could be assigned to prisons and reformatories. However, this solution created as many problems as it solved. The sponsors of an early twentieth-century New York legisla-tive bill were aware of these derivative problems when they called for the establish-ment of "a custodial asylum for feeble-minded male delinquents." Lewis (1912–1913) noted that this New York bill had been supported by penitentiary war-dens "who see their prisons and reformatories 'clogged' . . . with mentally backward and deficient prisoners, who . . . 'have no place in a reformatory in the first place, and are a hindrance to its work for the brighter boys' " (p. 10). The same point had been made years earlier by Allison (1904). Allison had warned that the typical prison had devolved into "an indiscriminate place of mere detention" where the "habitual criminal, the insane and defective are not sifted out from the general prison population" (pp. 292–293).

Changing Architecture

Throughout the nineteenth century, the public's fears had influenced the design and construction of the facilities to which persons with disabilities were assigned. Proponents of less oppressive styles of architecture were aware that this apprehension was widespread and genuine. Therefore, they expressed their thoughts in ways that would not startle readers. This careful style of rhetoric was reflected in one of the very early books on asylums. Samuel Tuke (1815a) was the author of this publication, which he originally had drafted as a letter to the administrators who were planning an asylum in New York. In that letter, Tuke had made remarks about an architect's drawing for a specialized facility that was under construction at Wakefield, England. Tuke's remarks revealed some of his assumptions about that facility and the disabled persons who would occupy it. At the time that he was writing, these assumptions were extremely progressive.

> I hope [the architectural drawing] will not be altogether useless. Should it be thought too expensive, I think the rooms, 1, 2, and 3, might be dispensed with, and rooms marked "*attendants, sick, and bath*," might be appropriated to the patients during the day. The attendants [*sic*] room is not a requisite, though it has been thought that it would be more agreeable to patients of superior rank to have the society of a servant. This, however, chiefly applied to the convalescents, and these might occupy the room marked '*sick*,' [*sic*] while the middle class, and the attendants, would be very suitably placed in the larger room in the centre, marked "attendants." [*sic*] (Emphasis in the original text, Tuke, 1815a, p. 6)

Samuel Tuke (1815a) noted that the Wakefield asylum had been designed as a single-level structure. However, he wrote that "if you are inclined for the sake of appearance, to make the centre building two stories high, you might bring the wings nearer to the centre and accommodate most of the convalescent patients with bed rooms [*sic*] in the upper story" (pp. 6–7). Tuke added that "in this case perhaps it would be desirable to give the wings a radiating form" (pp. 6–7). As a final caveat, he recommended that "the new asylum should be placed a few miles from the city" in order to encourage visits by the friends and families of the patients. Regarding the rationale for familial visits, Tuke explained that these visits were "so important for the welfare of asylums" that administrators should make the opportunity "as easy as it can be with propriety" (p. 8).

Samuel Tuke (1964) had published a report in 1814. In that early report, he had included illustrations of a three-story asylum at York, England. These pictures, which are reproduced as Figures 2.1 and 2.2, indicated that the York

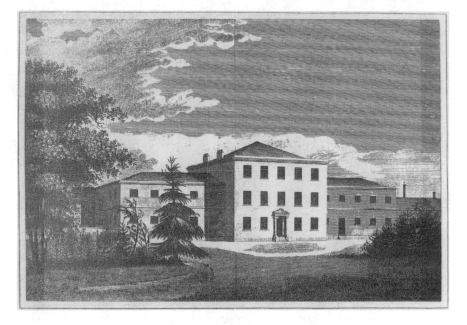

Figure 2.1. Illustration of an Early Nineteenth-Century British Asylum.

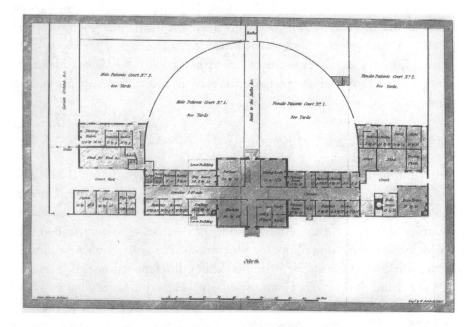

Figure 2.2. Illustration of the Interior of an Early Nineteenth-Century British Asylum.

asylum comprised small, personalized bedrooms. It also included carefully planned outdoor areas for the inmates' use. The desire to help the patients feel comfortable and respected was apparent in the features of another architectural drawing that Tuke (1815b) published a year later (Figure 2.3).

The past, current, and emerging beliefs of British citizens influenced the design and construction of custodial facilities. Their beliefs also influenced the design and construction of scholastic facilities. The resulting facilities assisted or hindered educational practitioners. William Holmes (1912) had made this point in an early twentieth-century report. In that document, he had described a model of assessment and intervention that clearly was constrained by the availability of suitable scholastic facilities.

> If a child in the regular primary school is thought to be mentally defective he is sent to the local special school for examination by the school physician. After the examination he is kept at the special school, for observation. After this probationary period he may be returned to the regular school as being a normal child, retained in the special school until the age of fourteen or sixteen, or dismissed from school altogether as too defective to profit by special school instruction. No provision is made for the care of this latter class of children except in poor-houses. (p. 12)

In his book, William Holmes (1912) had included architectural schemata of several schools that had been designed to complement the British philosophy of special education. These drawings, which are reproduced in Figure 2.4, are largely indistinguishable from the architectural drawings of the schools for students without disabilities. The only strikingly distinctive features of the special educational buildings were the workshops for manual training.

Changing American Architecture

Writing during the first quarter of the twentieth century, Anderson (1919) documented the negative attitudes that American citizens had displayed toward persons with disabilities. He focused his attention on the citizens of Georgia. To provide an historical context, Anderson alleged that Georgia's citizens had been ignoring persons with disabilities for generations. However, Anderson thought that the state leaders eventually began to exhibit different attitudes. He referred to a report from the Georgia Commission on Feeblemindedness that had been published during 1918. Anderson believed that this report had helped the legislators recognize "the serious consequences of the state's failure to provide proper care and training for this class of persons" (p. 527). With regard to those "serious

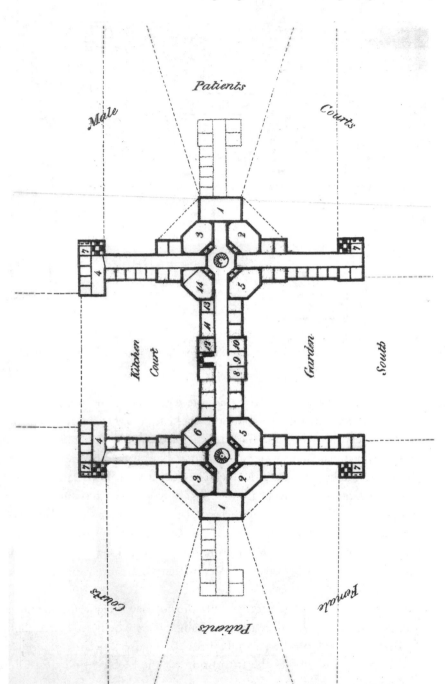

Figure 2.3. Illustration of the Interior and Grounds of an Early Nineteenth-Century British Asylum.

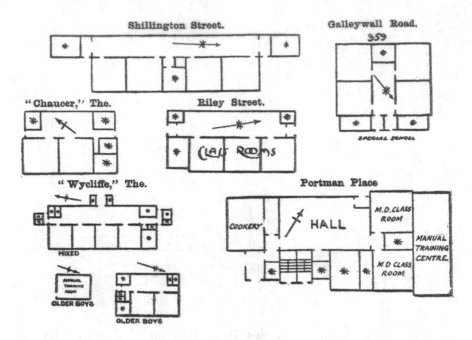

Figure 2.4. Early Twentieth-Century Special Education Facilities in Great Britain.

consequences," Anderson concluded that the legislators were not particularly struck by the suffering that disabled persons had endured. He thought that they were more impressed by the suffering that disabled persons inflicted on others. Anderson explained that "state-wide surveys, special investigations, and prolonged, painstaking, thoroughgoing scientific researches [*sic*] have demonstrated the positive and close relationship of feeblemindedness to many of society's most serious social problems" (p. 528). Some of the social problems that the legislators of Georgia linked to disabilities included crime, juvenile vice, prostitution, venereal disease, and pauperism. In the aftermaths of their epiphanies, the Georgia legislators assigned higher priority to the construction of state facilities for persons with disabilities.

In one of his reports, Anderson (1920) provided architectural schemata of American facilities at which children with disabilities were being educated. Some of these diagrams are reproduced in Figure 2.5, Figure 2.6, and Figure 2.7. Figure 2.5 depicts a building at the Institution for the Feeble-Minded in Ohio. Figure 2.6 illustrates a building at the Massachusetts School for the Feeble-Minded. Unlike those recently established British institutions that had been designed for daycare, the American facilities were intended for resident patients. Anderson also

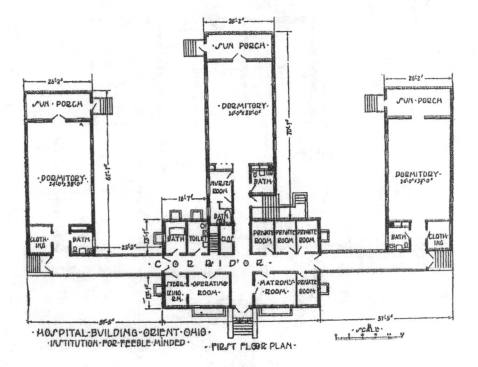

Figure 2.5. Early Twentieth-Century Special Education Facilities in Ohio.

included a diagram of a recreational building that was intended for the teachers, administrators, and professional staff at an asylum (Figure 2.7).

Anderson (1921) later published an historical account in which he detailed some of the changing perspectives from which the public and professionals had been viewing persons with disabilities. His editorialized remarks had clear implications for the types of facilities to which patients had been assigned during different eras.

> It was the hope of the early pioneers . . . to arouse the dormant faculties of the feebleminded. . . . For a period real enthusiasm existed over the possibilities in this plan of training, and the early schools were all purely educational in character. . . . When it became fully appreciated that feeblemindedness was incurable, that "once feebleminded always feebleminded," interest in the attempts to educate the feebleminded greatly diminished and public attention became centered upon another element of the problem, the heredity of the feebleminded. . . . Close upon these investigations came reports from state prisons, reformatories, workhouses, jails, houses of correction, and courts, showing the great frequency of feeblemindedness amongst juvenile delinquents, adult criminals, vagrants, prostitutes,

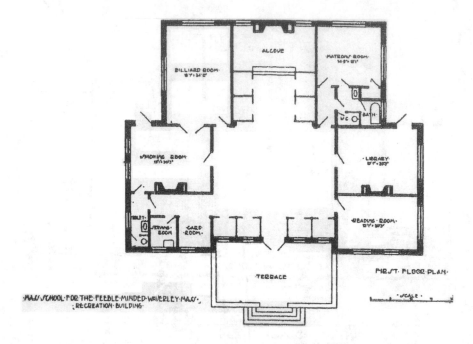

Figure 2.6. Early Twentieth-Century Special Education Facilities in Massachusetts.

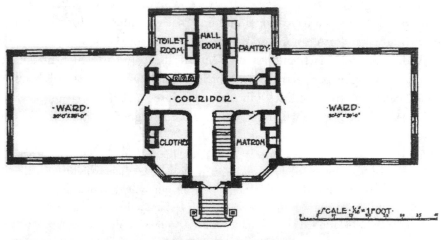

Figure 2.7. Early Twentieth-Century Recreational Facility for the Staff of an Asylum.

and the like. . . . There followed a period that may be called the custodial period, marked by the slogan: "Lifelong segregation or sterilization of all feebleminded persons." (pp. 91–92)

Anderson proclaimed that society was entering a new period in the way that it treated persons with disabilities. The progression into this new period struck Anderson as inevitable because the "permanent segregation or sterilization of all defectives, however good these theories may be, has been found to be impossible in the present state of public conscience" (p. 92). The emerging era, which would entail less restrictive alternatives, might include "state-wide supervision of all mental defectives" as well as "special-class training and after-care supervision" (p. 92).

Less Restrictive Facilities

Down (1876) was a nineteenth-century British physician who had chronicled the ways in which the treatment of persons with disabilities had changed. He was struck by how recently most of the significant changes had transpired. Downs observed candidly that "even so short a period as fifty years ago it would have been regarded as vain enthusiasm to expend care or thought on members of the community who were treated in every way was the solitary ones which their name suggests" (p. 5).

Daniel Tuke (1878; 1882; 1885) shared Down's views about the brutality with which persons with mental disabilities historically had been treated. Tuke detected this brutality in the stark and barren facilities to which disabled persons were assigned. He must have made his readers wince when he recapitulated the observations that had been made by the visitors to British asylums. For example, he quoted an eighteenth-century visitor who had cast his chilling observations into verse.

> For other views than these within appear,
>
> And Woe and Horror dwell for ever here;
>
> For ever from the echoing roofs rebounds
>
> A dreadful Din of heterogeneous sounds:
>
> From this, from that, from every quarter rise
>
> Loud shouts, and sullen groans, and doleful cries;
>
> With the chambers which this Dome contains,
>
> In all her 'frantic' forms, Distraction reigns:
>
> Rattling his chains, the wretch all raving lies,
>
> And roars and foams, and Earth and Heaven defies.
> (Anonymous, 1776, as quoted by Daniel Tuke, 1882, p. 75)

Daniel Tuke collated multiple observations from visitors to asylums. For example, he quoted remarks from one eighteenth-century physician who had reported that the patients "are ordered to be bled about the latter end of May, according to the weather" (T. Monroe, visiting physician at Bethlem Asylum, 1783, as quoted by Tuke, 1882, p. 79). This physician continued that "after they have been bled, they take vomits, once a week for a certain number of weeks; after that we purge the patients." Daniel Tuke adjured his readers to "condemn the lamentable ignorance and miserable medical red-tapism [*sic*] which marked the practice of lunacy in former times" (p. 80).

After he had compiled quotations from visitors to asylums, Daniel Tuke supplemented this collection with illustrations from visiting artists. He described one illustration that depicted "a maniac lying on straw in one of the cells" and on whom "there is a chain clearly visible" (1882, p. 73). Daniel Tuke described another illustration in which a patient "was secured by chains as there represented, consisting of (1) a collar, encircling the neck, and confined by a chain to a pole fixed at the head of the patient's bed, (2) an iron frame, the lower part of which encircled the body, and the upper part of which passed over the shoulders, having on either side apertures for the arms, which encircled them above the elbow; (3) a chain passing from the ankle of the patient to the foot of the bed" (p. 79). Figure 2.8, which appeared as the frontispiece to a book that Daniel Tuke's father had published in 1813 (Samuel Tuke, 1964), was typical of the illustrations to which Daniel Tuke had called attention.

The treatment of persons with disabilities improved during the late 1800s and the early part of the subsequent century. Duncan (1866) provided examples of nineteenth-century changes. He noted that some asylum staffs had begun to offer educational opportunities to their patients. Duncan recommended that the staff members at all institutions begin to offer educational classes to children with less severe disabilities. He suggested that children attend classes during the day and return to their homes at night. The daytime educational facilities he had in mind would be furnished with "a quiet place for out-of-door exercises," gymnastic equipment, "simple school materials for elementary instruction," and an "apparatus for the purpose of mechanical industry and amusement" (p. 89).

Although the treatment of persons with disabilities did improve, the inhumane conditions at asylums were not eliminated. Toward the end of the nineteenth century, Daniel Tuke (1892c) clearly made this point. After noting that the directors of a particular British asylum had been applauded for eliminating "mechanical" restraining devices, Tuke objected that those inhumane devices still were in place. He concluded that some of the public's impressions about recent improvements had been "quite a mistake" (p. 29).

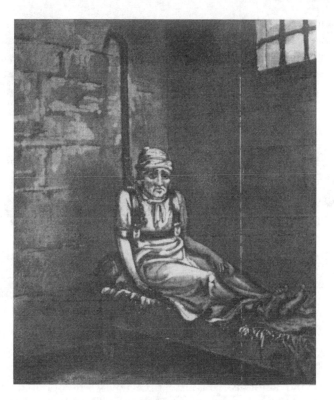

Figure 2.8. Depiction of Patient Abuse at a Nineteenth-Century British Asylum.

Less Restrictive American Facilities

Late nineteenth-century Americans began to search for alternatives to asylums. Some of them believed that alternative facilities were needed for humanitarian reasons. Others thought that they were necessary because the asylums were too expensive to construct and maintain. During this era, Knight presented a report to the Conference of Charities and Correction. In that 1892 report, he addressed those American citizens who had humanitarian concerns about asylums. Knight also addressed those with financial concerns. Knight addressed both issues by endorsing the development of facilities that enabled inmates to be productive. In the type of facilities that he had in mind, the inmates would discharge maintenance chores and supervise their fellow patients. Knight listed the humanitarian and practical advantages of his plan.

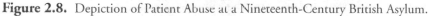

[Superintendents of asylums] have found that, even for money, it is difficult to get suitable people who are willing to come into contact with the lowest grade in the right spirit—a spirit which demands patience, cheerfulness, and affection. But they do find that what is called "the imbecile" will share his pleasures and attainments with his weaker brother with a sense of high privilege in being allowed to share it; that none makes tenderer [*sic*] care-takers nor, under supervision, more watchful ones; and that the bond of fellowship so engendered is of lasting benefit. This is why the colony plan recommends itself to us. (G. H. Knight, from a Report to the Nineteenth Conference of Charities and Correction, 1892, as quoted by Fernald, 1893, p. 218)

Seven years after Knight had made the preceding recommendations, Johnson (1899) reported about the progress in the establishment of communal homes for persons with disabilities. Johnson judged that facilities offering this type of care were "not in full operation anywhere" (p. 471). Despite this slow pace of development, Johnson believed that the experiments with communal homes had provided indisputable evidence of their value. He assured readers that this evidence "abundantly justified the expectations" of those who had been promoting communal living.

At the same time that the communes were helping adults with disabilities, the American public schools became the sites for experimental initiatives to help disabled children. By the end of the nineteenth century, the school administrators in several cities had begun to offer special educational services. Those scholars who were proponents of special education attempted to sway the public's attitudes through books, reports, and editorials. Of course, the scholars who opposed special education used the same tools to influence the public's attitudes. Writing at the beginning of the twentieth century, Waldemar Groszmann (1906) sided with those scholars who were pessimistic about the school-based programs. He bluntly advised his readers that it would be "impossible to obtain satisfactory results with atypical children in the public or private schools" (p. 442). However, unlike most opponents of special education, Groszmann did not believe that disabled children would fail because they were inherently uneducable or incorrigibly dangerous. Instead, Groszmann maintained that they would fail because so few teachers had been trained to meet the needs of special students. In addition to having doubts about the teachers, Groszmann also questioned the diagnostic procedures and the curricula that were prevalent.

Rather than simply criticize school-based programs, Groszmann (1906) proposed an alternative. He believed that a highly specialized type of education should be offered in conjunction with medical care. The paradigm for this new type of education would replicate the model that medical professionals already were employing.

Children [with disabilities] must be removed into an environment where perfect harmony and interaction exists between all influences. They require more than the school and home environments can offer. . . . Such careful treatment and equipment can be offered only by institutions especially adapted to the requirements of such work. Competent specialists, both in the fields of education and medicine, must co-operate in a study of each child's difficulties and needs. Such an institution must be, as it were, a psycho- and physiological laboratory for a scientific study of each case. In this way not only will each child receive the necessary observation, but data for a deeper study of the general problems will be obtained. (p. 442)

Hardy (1913), who was the Superintendent of the North Carolina School for the Feeble-Minded, did not discourage the building of asylums, special hospitals, and other restrictive facilities. In fact, he wrote that the first step in helping persons with disabilities was to establish additional facilities for those patients who were "urgently in need of permanent care" (p. 512). Despite his endorsement of asylums, Hardy thought that less restrictive facilities also were needed. He underscored the humanitarian and financial benefits of alternative facilities. For example, Hardy pointed out that "large colonies" could provide adult residents with the chance to "live as nearly a normal life as it is possible for them to live" (p. 512). With regard to facilities for disabled children, Hardy encouraged his colleagues to look to the schools. He encouraged them to replicate the special education programs that had been started in the public schools of New York City.

New Yorkers Use the Public Schools

The parents of children with disabilities demanded school-based programs. Their proactive efforts, as well as the school administrators' responses to those efforts, could be discerned throughout the first quarter of the twentieth century. Edson (1908), a New York superintendent, was quite aware of the political power that the parents wielded. He recommended that his fellow school administrators listen carefully to the parents and involve them in scholastic deliberations that would affect their children. Edson noted that the concerned parents hoped to promote school-based services that were similar to those in private schools. Edson wanted the public-school staffs to be responsive to these parents because some of them "cannot afford to meet the expenses involved in placing their children in private institutions, and are too proud or too indifferent to commit them to charitable institutions" (p. 351).

In reaction to the political pressure that the parents exerted, some school administrators did accept new responsibilities. Many of these responsibilities had been assumed exclusively by charitable institutions. Approving of this transition, Edson (1908) claimed that "no rivalry exists" between the administrators in the public schools and those in charitable institutions. He believed that the two groups would cooperate once their members realized that neither group by itself would be able to "care for all the unfortunate children in need of an education" (p. 351).

New York was one of the first cities in which school administrators began to offer special education. They were guided by the 1912 *School Inquiry Report on Ungraded Classes*, which had been written to strategically develop special services within the public schools of New York City. Farrell (1914a; 1914b; 1914c) quoted sections of this report, which included information about new types of educational facilities.

> Separate schools would . . . be established for [children with disabilities]. . . . The lowest grade cases, for whom little can be done, could be put in one group, and the teacher in charge would only be required to keep them happy, train them in simple habits, and do for them what their condition allows. Those who are a little higher could be put together in another class. . . . Ultimately these schools should develop into home schools, keeping the children as many hours as possible, and many of them even over night. And finally, they should develop into city institutions for defectives. (Passage from the *School Inquiry Report on Ungraded Classes*, 1912, as quoted by Farrell, 1914b, p. 57)

The authors of the *School Inquiry Report on Ungraded Classes* had suggested ways to provide special educational services to the children of New York City. Like these authors, Arthur Holmes (1915) endorsed public-school-based special education. Holmes even provided specific advice on the ideal location for special educational classrooms. For example, he recommended that the classrooms "should not be adjacent to other classrooms [*sic*], if possible, since the tramp of physical exercises, the noise of manual work, the sound of music and singing may entirely interfere with other classes" (p. 231). Holmes also insisted that "quiet, air, light, space, comfort and convenience" were "cardinal points in the location of the class-rooms [*sic*]" (p. 231).

In addition to giving advice about locations and dimensions for special educational classrooms, Holmes (1915) made recommendations about the optimal types of equipment with which to furnish them. He thought the selection of suitable materials was critical because children with disabilities "can not [*sic*] read and image as a normal child can; they must see, hear, taste, smell, handle in order to become acquainted with the strange and overwhelmingly complex world about them" (pp. 232–233). Discouraging the use of "store-bought" instructional items, Holmes preferred familiar and readily accessible objects. He suggested that teachers fill their classrooms with "pictures, flags, ferns, flowers, aquaria, birds, curios, samples of manufacturing products, [and] all the endless odds and ends that do make up the complex world about them" (p. 232). He added that that these items "should be where these children can see and handle the things themselves" (p. 232).

New Yorkers Experiment With Alternative Programs for Adults

During the first quarter of the twentieth century, the citizens of New York City had established special programs in their public schools. Some observers believed that these innovative programs provided unprecedented scholastic opportunities. Nonetheless, other observers focused on the liabilities that were associated with the programs. During the period that they were establishing the new programs for disabled children, the citizens of the state of New York also established innovative programs for adults with disabilities. As they had with the school-based programs, some persons detected liabilities within the alternative adult programs. For this reason, the advocates of alternative adult programs were extremely careful when they were explaining their initiatives.

Writing during World War I, Bowers (1917) had illustrated the cautious manner in which special educators conducted themselves. Bowers acknowledged that the advocates of asylums viewed persons with disabilities as serious threats. He was aware that the advocates of less restrictive forms of care held extremely different views. Bowers seemed to appeal to the group that was fearful when he assured readers that he personally was "devoid of maudlin sentiment" and concerned about protecting "the public from individuals who offend society and violate her laws" (p. 221). As for "the dangerous insane, the morally insane, the sexual perverts, and the habitual criminals," Bowers unquestionably reaffirmed the genuine threat that they posed. He suggested that these groups be "sent to hospitals for the criminal [*sic*] insane permanently or until a cure was affected [*sic*]" (p. 229).

Despite the harsh remarks that he had made about the treatment of persons who were "dangerous insane," Bowers (1917) demonstrated flexibility about the treatment of persons with less severe disabilities. He may have surprised the advocates of asylum-based care when he actually recommended alternative facilities as the most suitable sites for persons with mild and moderate disabilities. Bowers explained that he opposed the indiscriminate imprisoning of patients with mild and moderate disabilities because "society is being poorly protected when it sends insane and mentally defective individuals to penal institutions and then releases them uncured" (p. 221). On the basis of this conviction, Bowers endorsed facilities at which persons with mild and moderate disabilities would have a chance to be cured rather than merely detained.

Bernstein (1918; 1920), who was the superintendent of a New York asylum, spoke in favor of less restrictive facilities. Bernstein assumed that his readers would recognize the humanitarian benefits for the patients who were assigned to alternative facilities. However, he wondered whether the public realized the corollary benefits that accrued to society. Bernstein pointed to three ways in which society profited from alternative residence facilities. These facilities, which could be designed so that residents would be self-supporting, would help "the state financially" (1920, p. 2). Another advantage was that their inexpensiveness "permits of increased facilities." Finally, the patients at these facilities, many of whom could develop vocations, would add "to the community's supply of labor" (1920, p. 2).

To emphasize the feasibility of communal living, Bernstein (1920) recounted historical details of an "agricultural colony" that had spun off from the New York asylum that he managed.

> A supervisor and assistant matron . . . took possession of this farm, marching away from the old asylum premises, led by the patients' band, with a team and large sleigh, two cows, one extra horse, a few cooking utensils, one month's supply of food, and the eight patients' clothing and trunks. . . . Four more boys were placed on the farm soon afterwards, making twelve boys there, and this number was later increased to twenty. (pp. 2–3)

Although some citizens in the United States viewed Bernstein's experiment as a pioneering initiative, others realized that the Europeans had implemented successful programs of this type decades earlier.

Bernstein (1918; 1920) used the phrase "colonization programs" to describe those programs that provided group living arrangements for adults with disabilities. In addition to sanctioning these programs, Bernstein championed the practice of finding "extra-institutional" jobs for the participants in them. Bernstein had noted that the diversion of state funds to "colonization" programs had enabled the citizens of New York to meet the needs of more individuals than they could have met through institution-based care. Relying on the same logic, Bernstein argued that extra-institutional employment extended the scope of the colonization programs while simultaneously reducing their expenses.

Irrespective of whether patients were assigned to colonies or to extra-institutional jobsites, Bernstein (1920) thought that those patients should generate a portion of the budget that was needed to sustain them. He recommended that female patients engage in "domestic work, hand laundry, and sewing" (p. 26). He recommended that the males assume responsibilities on "various parcels of state-owned land and on abandoned or undeveloped parcels of state-owned land and on abandoned or undeveloped farms" (pp. 26–27).

In an article that he had written in the early 1920s, Bernstein (1923) referred to the extra-institution supervision of individuals with disabilities as "parole care." As in many of his other reports, Bernstein emphasized that this practice was economical. The recognition of these monetary benefits had led "the state of New York not only to continue the work, but to extend it rapidly" (p. 444). Although Bernstein continually stressed sound financial management, his humanitarian principles were quite discernible.

> From one-third to one-half of all the mentally defective persons who need state care can be provided for under a reasonable system of colony and parole care and supervision. . . . What many of these social misfits and mentally disturbed patients need is not lock-ups and custodial institutions and prisons—or even hospitals . . . but rather a change of environment. They need, not the restraining influence of high walls and iron enclosures and guards, but rather the sustaining, diverting, and comforting influence of a simple, comfortable home . . . where their energies can find an outlet in useful, healthful work suited to their capacities. (pp. 470–471)

Bernstein (1923) warned the administrators at communal homes that the hiring of appropriately qualified supervisors would be difficult. In spite of the challenges, he adjured them to be persistent in their searches for ideally qualified supervisors. Bernstein advised them that the ideal supervisor would be "a house mother with sympathy and insight bred of experience" (p. 471).

Massachusetts Citizens Experiment With Communal Facilities

The citizens of Massachusetts had established a "parole" system of care during the first quarter of the twentieth century. Gegenheimer (1948) examined historical records, reports, and letters in order to better understand this program. Even though the parole program had not been established formally until 1922, it had been initiated on an experimental basis a decade earlier. Gegenheimer recounted some details from that early period.

> In 1912, Dr. Fernald at Waverley first commented in his annual report on the fact that certain patients were being released from the institution to go home on trial. In cases where the authorities were unwilling to discharge the patients but had no power to compel custody, they allowed them to go, with the plan that they report in person at the School at regular intervals. Dr. Fernald felt that this informal after-care should be extended and put on a permanent basis. (p. 92)

After she had examined the records associated with this initiative, Gegenheimer concluded that it had been established "chiefly in response to requests of relatives" (p. 92).

Shuttleworth and Potts (1922), who were members of Britain's Commission on the Care and Control of the Feeble-minded, had toured some of the American facilities for persons with disabilities. Without elaborating further, they noted "the economical character of the buildings" in which care was provided. Although they were impressed by the traditionally managed facilities, Shuttleworth and Potts were impressed just as much by some of the alternative facilities, such as the "industrial colonies for permanent care." Despite the fact that they documented only several alternative facilities, they characterized them as "essential" components of the American system.

To help their readers understand the daily routines of the patients who were assigned to alternative facilities, Shuttleworth and Potts (1922) reproduced a section of a report that had been written by a visitor.

> [The residents] are all required to do manual work, and many of them do nearly the full work of a free labourer [*sic*]. We saw a group of four, with heavy sledges and hammers, breaking rock and drilling it for blasting with explosives. They were working steadily and without supervision. Farther on was another group of five men working in a field. They were bringing in stooks of corn, which they were loading upon a cart. Others in the shed were unloading and storing the corn. A further group was hauling bricks in wheelbarrows. At a little distance there was a row of about a dozen, who, under the supervision of one man only, were working a field with sharp pickaxes. An imbecile was ploughing with a pair of horses, his daily task [*sic*]. (Passage from a report by the Commission on the Care and Control of the Feeble-minded, n.d., as quoted by Shuttleworth & Potts, 1922, p. 38)

Shuttleworth and Potts observed that the preceding notes had been made by an observer who had visited the Templeton Colony for Feeble-Minded Males. They explained that this was an alternative facility in Massachusetts.

Urban Communal Facilities Emerge

Many of the advocates for less restrictive facilities had recommended that adult males labor on farms. They recommended that females assume domestic jobs at communal residences. One of the advantages of these plans was the relative ease with which they could be implemented. However, some analysts believed that these suggestions were too conservative. For example Curtis (1924) believed that adults with disabilities could become successful factory workers. He buttressed his proposal with psychological and anecdotal information.

> The whole tendency of efficiency reorganization . . . is to reduce each process to a single motion, endlessly repeated by each worker. Such work requires a feeble-minded

worker. . . . Ford says he can use several thousand feeble-minded in his factory, pay them six dollars a day, and have them earn the money. (p. 643)

Curtis (1924) was convinced that workforces could be formed from disabled individuals who lived adjacent to factories. In a chilling scenario, he described the circumstances under which the laborers could marry and maintain families.

Where one member of a couple consents to sterilization, the couple should be allowed to marry. The colony would soon get over its fear, and marriage might become the mode. They would still lack one feature of the normal family, the child. But they might, under close supervision, adopt or borrow certain feeble-minded children from the institutions. (p. 644)

Financial and humanitarian considerations may have curtailed the full implementation of the plans that Curtis (1924) and like-minded colleagues had devised. However, more and more members of the public became receptive to innovative recommendations. They believed that disabled adults should have opportunities to live in their communities, discharge meaningful tasks, and interact with the general public. In a book aimed at teachers and school administrators, Scheidemann (1931) confirmed that the public's attitudes on these issues were shifting. The emergence of new attitudes toward disabled adults facilitated the development of novel treatments. Scheidemann believed that they also had facilitated a "present movement toward the de-institutionalization of school children" (p. ix). During the following decade, these changing attitudes became even more evident. The political movements that accompanied the changing attitudes also became more evident.

Regressive American Attitudes

During the early years of the twentieth century, some Americans had detected a more progressive approach to asylum management. After chronicling some of the changes at the asylum where he personally worked, Johnstone (1909a) concluded that this transformation was substantive. Furthermore, he believed that it already had improved the lives of the institutionalized patients. Even though Johnstone was personally gratified at this progress, he realized that many members of the public were unaware of it. As a result, they continued to criticize asylums.

I wonder if we who live in institutions ever take the trouble to find out what other people think about institutions? It is surprising to learn what the average intelligent man or woman who never has visited an institution believes it to be. Persons

just below the average, a large number of persons among the voters, think that institutions are places of bars and bolts and gloom and sorrow and sadness. (p. 124)

Writing in the early 1920s, Anderson (1921) shared Johnstone's assessment of
the positive changes that were taking place within American asylums. Although he
recognized the cruel manner in which disabled persons had been treated historically, Anderson proclaimed that a new era of care and treatment was beginning. The
changes to which Johnstone and then Anderson had referred eventually did transpire. Nonetheless, they did not take place as rapidly or as extensively as the two
scholars had concluded. In fact, multiple reports from that era proved that their
assessments had been unreasonably optimistic.

Negative attitudes toward persons with disabilities could be discerned after
World War I. Sometimes these attitudes were based on extremely regressive views.
One of Anderson's contemporaries provided an example of these negative attitudes.
The individual in this case had recommended the enactment of special immigra-
tion laws as a means of restricting persons with disabilities.

> The tests made at Ellis Island are insufficient to exclude inadequate germ plasm
> [*sic*]. The law permits deportation of aliens who prove defective within five years
> of admission to the country. It would help if the period within which deporta-
> tion might occur might be increased to ten or more years. Still better would it be
> if defectives or the potentially insane were turned back at Ellis Island and better
> still if they could be detected before starting on their journey to America.
> (Davenport, 1920, p. 178–179)

In the early 1920s, Anderson (1921) had announced the beginning of a new era
in the ways that persons with disabilities were being treated. Clearly, Davenport (1920),
who had written the preceding passage, had a different point of view. Many contemporaries agreed with Davenport. For decades, their negative views were evident. For
example, they were discernible in the initial sentence of a statute that was introduced
into the 1936 session of the Kentucky legislature (Arnold, 1936).

> Whenever the Superintendent or Warden of the State's reformatories or hospitals for
> the insane or feeble-minded shall be of the opinion that it is for the best interest of
> the patient or inmate and society that any inmate of the institution under his care
> should be sexually sterilized, such superintendent or warden is hereby authorized to
> cause to be performed by some capable physician or surgeon the operation of sterili-
> zation on any patient or inmate confined in such institution affected with insanity,
> idiocy, imbecility, feeble-mindedness, or epilepsy. (Passage from a statute introduced
> into the Kentucky state legislature, 1936, as quoted by Arnold, 1936, p. 220)

The authors of the preceding bill had seen it as a measure that would improve "the physical, mental, neural, or psychic condition of the inmate" (passage from a statue introduced into the Kentucky state legislature, 1936, as quoted by Arnold, 1936, p. 221). At the same time, they had displayed alarmingly regressive attitudes. In fact, they admitted that they had designed their bill to "protect society from the menace of procreation by said inmate" (passage from a statue introduced into the Kentucky state legislature, 1936, as quoted by Arnold, 1936, p. 221).

Preparing Teachers

Throughout the nineteenth century, scholars, educators, and citizens feared that the number of persons with disabilities was increasing. Twentieth-century citizens continued to express these fears. Writing during World War I, Bernstein (1917) had gathered information from "authorities" in order to clarify the problem. He focused his attention on the impressions of New York state authorities about the number of disabled persons in their state. Bernstein reported that these "authorities agree that there are approximately 32,000 feebleminded, or one in every 300 people, throughout the State of New York" (p. 201). The authorities believed that 6,000 disabled individuals had been assigned to institutions specifically "designed for them." They claimed that another 6,000 persons had been "confined in institutions not intended for their care" (p. 201). Bernstein added ominously that the remaining 20,000 disabled persons remained "at large in the community" (pp. 201–202). Bernstein assumed that these data would persuade his readers that the problem was grave. He hoped that they also would persuade readers to designate schools as sites at which disabled persons would receive care.

Proponents of school-based care believed that they had located the ideal facilities for students with disabilities. After all, schools were relatively cheap to construct. They could accommodate many more children than the asylums could handle. They already had staff members who had been trained to handle children with physical and emotional problems.

School-based care also was attractive because of its effectiveness, which had been demonstrated in Europe. Many European scholars had written testimonials about the positive impact of their programs. Berry (1909), who was a medical officer assigned to the British schools, had written about London's school-based programs for disabled children. He identified the typical participant in these programs as a student who "not being imbecile, and not being merely dull and backward, is by reason of mental defect incapable of receiving proper benefit from the instruction in an ordinary public elementary school" (p. 333). Berry emphasized that this type of student could "benefit from instruction in a certified special class or school" (p. 333).

Temperaments Required by Special Educators

Some experts thought that special educators required extraordinary temperaments. Seguin (1878) was an influential pioneer in special education. He had suggested that women might have the ideal temperaments to be successful special educators. After reminiscing about several females who had worked effectively in asylums, he observed that "none know today what women can do, and will aspire to" (p. 61). Seguin added that "it is no man's business for man to say they will do this or that; but we can advise and help them in the departments of our common work, when they have shown decided ability, by assisting them in adding knowledge to it" (p. 61).

Edson (1908), a New York City superintendent, also had firm convictions about the temperaments of special educators. He believed that each special educator "should be possessed of an even and sunny temperament, infinite patience, tact and firmness, great resourcefulness, and an intense human sympathy" (p. 353). As for more formal types of pedagogical preparation, Edson only recommended that special educators "should be specially trained for the work if possible, should be familiar with the literature on the subject, and by frequent visitation to other schools and institutions be reasonably familiar with what is going on in schools" (p. 354).

Writing in Great Britain, Lapage (1911) addressed his remarks to school administrators. He did not assume that special education was the peculiar purview of females. He pointed out that "it is, of course, necessary that one should be able to trust the men to whom one hands over such children" (p. 280). In a succinct description of the types of teachers who would be effective in special education classrooms, Lapage wrote that "they should be good-tempered and patient and willing to teach; careful also that the children do not get over-fatigued or wet and cold" (p. 280).

Skills Required by Special Educators

Some experts questioned whether the presence of warm and caring temperaments would enable teachers to instruct students with disabilities. They suggested that the teachers acquire specific knowledge and skills. For example, some experts believed that the special education teachers should possess a rudimentary understanding of psychology. In a book that they had published in 1900, two British educators (Collar & Crook, 1905) had called attention to the educational relevance of psychology. They pointed out that "in time past it was considered that the chief, and indeed almost the only, qualification necessary in a teacher was a knowledge [*sic*] of the subject to be taught" (p. v). Although they disagreed with persons who maintained this traditional attitude, they were just as worried by those experts who had begun to assign disproportionate importance to psychology. The British educators noted that "the tendency of the present day is to go to the other extreme, and regard a knowledge [*sic*] of psychology as being the only qualification that a teacher should bring to his work" (p. v).

Preston Search (1905), who was an American educator, went a step further than Collar and Crook (1905) had gone. Search agreed with his British colleagues about the advantages of professionally trained teachers. However, Search stressed the importance of establishing the types of environments that would enable trained teachers to be effective. He insisted that educators work under optimal conditions. For example, he recommended that each teacher instruct no more than 24 students. Although he fiercely defended this proposal, Search conceded that it would be extremely expensive to implement.

> The cost for teachers, increased by reduction of schools to twenty-four children, which is eminently desirable, and by the employment of better teachers, would be greater. But, after all, what are we living for if not for our children? Why does the wage-earner toil day after day, and the capitalist store up his money, if it is not to confer wealth upon the children? And what wealth is there that can for a moment be compared with glorious health, and the developing power which comes from a well-trained mind? (p. 103)

Although the preceding passage revealed Search's ardor, it may have had limited appeal to budget-minded administrators and school-board members.

Johnstone (1908) was another educational scholar who saw the value of pedagogical training. He encouraged the educators who were assigned to special classrooms to enroll in courses about children with disabilities. However, Johnstone believed that all elementary-school teachers, including those who worked in regular classrooms, would benefit from this coursework. Johnstone based this advice on the high probability that all teachers would encounter disabled children in their classrooms.

> No primary teacher thruout [*sic*] all the country but has had [*sic*] at least one mentally deficient child in her class. She has not been equipped to recognize him and so she has suffered much wear and tear on her nerve force and many an unfortunate child has been misused . . . because it was not understood. Our state normal schools will be greatly at fault if they do not at once make it their business to teach their students to know something of mental deficiency. (p. 1116)

More and more American scholars agreed that special educators needed to acquire specific knowledge and skills. This knowledge would enable them to meet the needs of children with mental problems. Williams (1909) believed that they also should be taught to help students with emotional problems. Williams then recommended that these elite instructors, whom he referred to as "competent teachers," should be assigned to "proper wards and out-patient clinics" (p. 198). Williams added that the highly specialized types of facilities that he had in mind were to "be provided, at least in every city" (p. 198). Two years later, Arthur Holmes (1911) judged that "most of the larger institutions of learning" had designated psychology as the basis for "the preparation of the teacher for more efficient professional work" (p. 11). Holmes applauded the professionally trained teachers who were graduating from these institutions. He assured them that they would be able to deal with a broad range of classroom problems, including "the investigation of the mental development of school children" (p. 11).

Van Sickle, Witmer, and Ayres (1911) wrote that special education teachers required "knowledge of expert methods of encouraging normal mental development" (p. 67). At the same time that they were making this recommendation about the preparation of teachers, Van Sickle, Witmer, and Ayres conceded that their advice would be difficult to implement. They explained that the knowledge they had in mind would be hard to acquire because "there is not one institution which offers all of the varied training which a teacher of exceptional children may require" (p. 67).

Van Sickle, Witmer, and Ayres (1911) had referred to the difficulty of finding an institution of higher learning at which special educators could acquire knowledge and training. Clearly, university administrators had to change their views of special educators and accept the responsibility for preparing them. However, even if the university administrators cooperated, Van Sickle, Witmer, and Ayres predicted that their plan would fail. They noted that the cost of employing this new type of personnel would be prohibitive.

> It would be a mistake for [the superintendent] to wait until he has ascertained the whole number of backward or of physically and otherwise exceptional children, and then attempt to introduce a complete organization to meet the needs of all. The number of such children will be found to be much larger than the superintendent has dreamed; the expense will be much greater than the school board will be likely to assume in connection with a new enterprise in education. Moreover it would be impossible to find anywhere in the United States a sufficient number of adequately trained teachers to meet the needs of the large number of different types of exceptional children. (p. 66)

Not all scholars encouraged the placement of children with disabilities in the public-schools. Van Sickle, Witmer, and Ayres (1911) had anticipated that the cost of this initiative, even though it was much less expensive than asylum-based care, was too high for many schools districts to consider. They also recognized the force of the other arguments from the opponents of school-based care. These opponents had judged that children with disabilities were unable to genuinely profit from any type of education. They alleged that students with disabilities were too immoral to be placed in the schools. Some of them thought the students were too dangerous for the schools.

Binet and Simon (1914), who were European psychologists, identified another obstacle to special education. After making observations about the spread of school-based special education programs in France, they warned proponents to "be prepared . . . for the hostility of the school staff" (p. 48). To underscore their point, Binet and Simon gave examples of ways in which a hostile school administrator could undermine the efforts to educate children with disabilities.

> It may be that [the school administrator] is indifferent, or does not believe in special education, or simply does not choose to put himself about, or, again, he may be timid and afraid of trouble, or may shrink from the recriminations of parents, behind whom he sees the hostile shadow of some town councilor or journalist. Lastly, he may be an ignoramus who, even at this time of day, imagines that a child cannot be a defective unless he has incontinence of urine or a sugar-loaf head. (p. 49)

Binet and Simon had called attention to the ways in which school administrators and nonspecial educators might restrict the instruction of children with disabilities. Their remarks turned out to be remarkably prescient.

Training Special Educators

Within an early account of American special education, Lincoln (1903) had described the ways in which Boston's school administrators had appointed special educators. Lincoln indicated that the administrators hired "the best possible teachers," whom they judged to be women with "experience in their profession" and knowledge of "kindergarten methods" (p. 84). Although the school administrators eventually were able to hire several experienced special teachers, they were unable to attract the full number that they required. Therefore they began to provide some of their recent recruits with three-month-long internships.

The school administrators and the members of Boston's board of education had concluded that special education teachers required appropriate training. Formal courses and supervised internships could provide that training. Training seemed especially important because neither the administrators nor their board members understood the precise way in which disabled students should be instructed. As such, they could not state their expectations for the instructors that they were hiring. Lincoln, who was aware of this problem, observed that "the teachers thus chosen were practically allowed to act as their own judgment dictated" (1903, p. 84).

Chace (1904) was convinced that professionally prepared special educators had value. He stated firmly that these "teachers should have special training for their work" (p. 390). Like many others, Chace did recognize that the opportunities for special education training were limited. He therefore gave advice to school administrators about some ways to secure this training for their staffs. For example, he recommended that they send their staffs to formal programs, such as the six-week training program at the New Jersey Training School for Feeble-minded Boys and Girls. Chace also praised the expedient teacher-training procedures that the school administrators of Boston had implemented.

Training Programs in New York City

Like the administrators in the Boston school district, New York City's school administrators had been searching for special educators. Farrell (1908–1909), who was the director of special education, wrote about the difficulties she had recruiting teachers in New York City. Farrell judged that the initial shortage of qualified personnel was so acute that it became the chief limitation on the growth of New York City's special education programs. She lamented that New York City had enough children with disabilities to justify the development of a model system of care and education. Demonstrating her political sophistication, she added that New York City also befitted from the leadership by a superintendent who was "the greatest public school man in this country" (p. 95). She concluded that the City's programs were suffering because "we have not teachers enough to fill the great need of the schools" (p. 95). To solve this problem, the New York City Board of Education approved a plan in which those teachers who volunteered to work with disabled learners would receive "three months' leave of absence, with full pay for the purposes of study. . . . in a school or institution for the trainnig of mentally deficient children" (p. 95).

Farrell (1914b) later provided additional details about the difficulty she had arranging professional training. She reminisced that in 1906 "an effort was made to have certain of the best institutions for the feebleminded devise means of training teachers for service in the public schools" (p. 65). However, the staffs were unresponsive. In 1910 and 1911, she repeated her supplications to the professors. Although the faculty members at the Brooklyn Training School for Teachers eventually did establish a teacher preparation program, Farrell felt that they should have been more professional. Because these faculty members already had devised a program to prepare employees for asylums, they decided to use asylums at the internship sites for the public-school trainees. Farrell scolded them for failing to provide the public-school trainees with "conditions similar to those under which they must work" (p. 65).

Other educators repeated Farrell's allegations about the unwillingness of the administrators at New York City's postsecondary institutions to train special educators. For example, Maennel (1909) specifically addressed this point. He wrote that "except for the summer course for teachers at the Vineland Training School [in New Jersey], and a special course on the Education of Defectives at the New York University School of Pedagogy, there is no means of training teachers for work among exceptional children" (p. 240).

Maennel (1909) had referred to the special education courses at the Vineland Training School. Johnstone (1909a), who was an administrator at that institution, commented on the student-centered philosophy of instruction to which the teachers in these courses were exposed. He explained that "we measure everything by the amount of [student] happiness we get out of it, or how much happiness we lose by doing it" (p. 125). He described several features of this summer program.

> Dr. Goddard has a course of lectures and much laboratory work that the teachers are required to do. They have one hour each day in the school rooms teaching various lines. There are two periods a week in which . . . the principal . . . teaches them the elements of various lines of industrial work. . . . The principal gives a period each day where practical work of the school room is discussed and methods taken up. (p. 125)

Smart (1908), who was a physician assigned to the schools, confirmed that New York City lacked qualified special educators. She added that it also lacked opportunities for training additional personnel. She advised school administrators to resolve the "burning question" about "how our work is to progress without properly equipped teachers" (p. 1144). However, Smart thought it was just as important to resolve "how teachers are to be properly trained without access to special schools or classes for this particular purpose" (p. 1144).

Because they could not locate qualified special educators, many school administrators had hired untrained instructors. Convinced that the untrained teachers had been ineffective, Smart (1908) applauded the enactment of a New York City regulation that required written and oral tests before special education teaching licenses would be awarded. However, this requirement had tightened the bottleneck though which the supply of teachers had to pass. Smart explained that "thirty or forty individuals may enter an examination for license to teach" children with disabilities but that only 25 percent of the applicants would "pass the preliminary theoretic, written test" (p. 1144). She continued that "out of this small percentage not more than three of four [would] be able to stand the practical, oral test" (p. 1144). Because such a small percentage of applicants could meet the licensing standards, some school administrators and aspiring teachers had recommended that licensing standards be relaxed. Smart offered a different solution; she wanted to establish additional training programs.

Smart (1908) had pointed out that the establishment of new teacher preparation programs would provide additional training opportunities. She encouraged the faculty for these new programs to set high standards. Like her professional colleagues, Smart did not conceal her disapproval of New York City's current programs. For example, she was displeased that New York University's training courses were "still in the constructive state and only partially doing their work" (p. 1143). Although she did approve of the program at the Vineland Training School, Smart still fumed because it was "only held for a few weeks in the summer" (p. 1143).

The opportunities to enroll in special educational courses eventually did increase. Nonetheless, the total number of opportunities remained inadequate. As a result, many untrained and unqualified teachers were assigned to special education classrooms. Maennel (1909) provided some practical tips for these teachers. For example, he counseled them about the number of students that they should admit into their classrooms. As a point of reference, Maennel referred to an 1894 decision in which the Prussian Minister of Education had limited the size of all classes to 25 students. However, Maennel thought that a class of 25 special students still would be inappropriate, especially in the lower grades. He suggested that 15 students was a more realistic limit.

During the early years of the twentieth century, the supply of trained educators had not been adequate to meet the needs of the large urban school districts. This shortage was documented even in communities such as New York City and Boston, which comprised colleges with prominent teacher preparation programs. Farrell (1914b) reported data that confirmed the gravity of this situation. The data came from the 1912 *School Inquiry Report on Ungraded Classes*, which had been drafted to guide the strategic expansion of special education in New York City. The authors of this report had highlighted weaknesses and strengths among that school district's special education staff. Regarding weaknesses, they noted that some of New York's special education teachers had been "inadequately trained." With unflinching candor, they stated that these untrained teachers had been providing instruction that was "seldom satisfactory" (passage from the *School Inquiry Report on Ungraded*

Classes, 1912, as quoted by Farrell, 1914b, p. 61). Even though they censured some members of New York City's instructional staff, the reporters praised other teachers. For example, they pointed out that 114 of New York City's 224 special educators had pursued "graduate study" at respected institutions. These institutions included New York University, the Vineland Training School, Adelphi College, and the College of the City of New York.

The panelists who had assembled the *School Inquiry Report on Ungraded Classes* gave several suggestions for increasing the supply of trained special educators. Some of their suggestions were straightforward. For example, they recommended that school administrators take steps "as rapidly as possible to provide training classes for teachers of defectives" (passage from the *School Inquiry Report on Ungraded Classes*, 1912, as quoted by Farrell, 1914b, p. 62). However, the authors were extremely realistic when they were analyzing the reasons for the New York City's current personnel problems. This realism was apparent when they acknowledged that some of those persons who aspired to be special educators had become discouraged by "difficult and arduous" coursework. The authors did not suggest a solution for this problem.

Awarding Bonuses to Special Educators

Some educational administrators used bonuses to lure special educators. The authors of the *School Inquiry Report on Ungraded Classes* believed that this strategy could increase the number of special educators in New York City. They recapitulated details of New York City's current reward system.

> The teacher of the ungraded class, who comes properly qualified, [is] to receive a bonus of $100 the first year, $200 the second, $300 the third, and so on, until it becomes $500—this in addition to the regular salary of the grade teacher. (Passage from the *School Inquiry Report on Ungraded Classes*, 1912, as quoted by Farrell, 1914b, p. 62)

Even though they supported New York City's use of financial incentives, the report's authors acknowledged that the meager amounts of the bonuses had failed to lure additional special educators.

The *School Inquiry Report on Ungraded Classes* was published in 1912. At the beginning of the 1920s, many school administrators still were concerned about the scarcity of trained special educators. Writing about Missouri's shortage, Wallin (1921b) proposed that state officials provide an annual stipend of $750.00 to each special educator. This stipend would supplement the salary that the educator was receiving from the school district. Wallin recommended that the Missouri officials would pay the stipend only if "this amount does not exceed two-thirds of the salary paid by the local board, provided the teacher has been especially trained for the particular type of child she has been employed to teach, and provided the classes have been approved by the state superintendent" (pp. 447–448). To clarify his references to teacher preparation, Wallin added that "the required preliminary training for certified teachers in all of the types of special classes is at least a two year's course in a standard normal school or college, and, in addition, not less than eight semester hours' credit in courses especially designed to prepare them for the particular type of work which they would do" (p. 448).

Wallin (1921b) initially had believed that bonuses would entice trained special educators. However, he later changed his mind. In an article that he wrote a decade after proposing the Missouri incentives, Wallin (1931) reviewed the disappointing consequences of the bonus program that school administrators in Baltimore had initiated.

> The public-school system of Baltimore has for several years provided a differential of $400 a year to special-class teachers having thirty semester hours of credit in approved courses in special education. However, a survey . . . showed that the regulation had remained wholly inoperative. Not a single teacher had received any increase beyond the initial bonus of $100, which was given without qualification. (Wallin, 1931, p. 607)

Wallin explained that Baltimore's school administrators, who had been willing to honor their financial commitments, were not to be blamed for this failure. The reason that they had not awarded the full amount of the bonuses was that "no teacher had earned the thirty hours of credit in courses in special education required for the additional $300 increment" (Wallin, 1931, p. 607).

The Public Pressures Educators

Critics were disgruntled about the schools. These critics included the parents who were dissatisfied with special education. The parents became dissatisfied when their children did not receive special educational services. Sometimes their children did not receive services because they lived in school districts without special education. At other times their children did not receive services because they lived in districts that could accommodate only a portion of the students who were eligible for special education.

Some parents of children with disabilities were especially difficult to appease. They exerted pressure on school administrators even after their children had been assigned to special education classes. The parents were annoyed if those classes were staffed by unqualified teachers. They also were annoyed by procedural issues. For example, the predictably slow progress of exceptional learners created administrative problems when the ages of the students disqualified them for services that they still needed.

Ayres (1911) was sympathetic to the parents who wished to retain their children in the schools for longer-than-typical periods. To place this problem in context, he noted that "about five years ago American educators awoke to a startled realization that a large proportion of all the children in the public schools were above the normal ages for their grades" (p. 657). After examining the records of more than 200,000 children in 29 cities, Ayres concluded that 17 percent of the children were not in the grades appropriate for their ages. They had been delayed because of late entrance to school, slow progress, or a combination of these two factors. Ayres insisted that all of those children who had been delayed because of slow progress should be retained until they had mastered essential skills. However, Ayres recognized that his suggestion would exacerbate the shortage of special educators. Were it to be implemented, this suggestion also would expand the total cost of education. Although it may have pleased parents, his suggestion must have incensed those businesspersons, politicians, and members of the public who had been urging the schools to operate with industry-like efficiency (Giordano, 2000; 2003; 2004; 2005).

Helping Neophyte Teachers

Peeved at those school administrators who had not hired special educators, parents pressured them to take action. Many of the administrators responded by hiring untrained and novice teachers. Predictably, the parents remained unsatisfied. They demanded teachers who could compete with the specialists in privately managed schools.

Educational experts recognized the expedient manner in which many school administrators had staffed their special education programs. Therefore, they began to give practical advice to the new teachers. For example, Thomas (1905) focused his attention on learning to read, for which he recommended that teachers employ phonics and kinesthetic activities. Thomas discouraged the teachers from requiring the memorization of sight words. Even though he had endorsed specific reading methods, the insightful Thomas was convinced that these methods were not inherently more effective than the others that were available. Assuming an open-minded perspective, he counseled teachers that "a little careful study of each child will show in which direction help is to be sought" (p. 385).

Devereux (1909) filled a book with pedagogical advice for inexperienced special educators. Devereux was a French educator who reminisced about strategies that she personally had found helpful. She wrote metaphorically that the secret of her success had involved the identification of "a 'peg' on which to hang the real mental training" that transpired in the classroom. Devereux explained that she had practical activities in mind. She counseled novice teachers that woodwork, basketry, and sewing could serve as effective mental pegs. She assured them that practical activities of this sort could be "a means of awakening the child" (p. 46).

Morgan (1914) was another educator who provided extremely practical information to instructors. For example, she gave them advice about some ingenious techniques for teaching students to count. Morgan told the instructors to worry less about the individual problem at hand and more about its underlying cause, which she believed was "always an ill-established associative connection" (p. 252). She added that students' learning problems were compounded when their teachers employed inappropriate pedagogical approaches and activities. Morgan was especially critical of drills-based mathematical activities, which she believed created student fatigue. She looked forward to an era when special educators would "understand every child's mental structure" and direct their interventions "to the fortifying of [each student's] weak points and the development of his tendencies" (p. ix).

Arthur Holmes (1915) recognized that most of the teachers who had been assigned to special education classrooms had not been formally prepared for their new responsibilities. He thought that even those instructors who had prior experiences in asylums would have to demonstrate the "widest latitude" of "invention and ingenuity" if they wished to become effective teachers. To reduce future personnel problems, Holmes recommended a distinctive model of teacher training. He thought that the "fitting of a special teacher for her work should be acquired in a school or college devoted to teaching teachers of public schools rather than one devoted to teaching teachers in institutions for the feeble-minded" (p. 225). Holmes predicted that prospective instructors would be attracted to this sophisticated type of training and the careers for which it prepared them. Holmes wrote poetically that prospective teachers would be lured by "the evident need of the children, the novelty and freedom of the field, the daily sight of appreciably growing boys and girls, the personal pride generated in each pupil as he responds to the training . . . the increasing expansion of the work throughout the world, [and] the constant and unceasing development of the teacher herself" (p. 229). In addition to these idealistic incentives, Holmes reminded prospective special educators that they would be rewarded with "extra recompense in salary" (p. 229).

During the nineteenth century, appropriate facilities and qualified teachers were in short supply. Because these problems were severe and pervasive, some parents and relatives of persons with disabilities personally had assumed educational responsibilities. In fact, many of them had assumed all of the responsibilities for social, vocational, and academic instruction. During the course of the twentieth century, the supply of professionally trained teachers increased. However, some specialists encouraged the parents and family members to supplement the work of the teachers. Wright (1915), who was the founder of a private school for deaf children, enthusiastically propounded this viewpoint. In his book, *What the Mother of a Deaf Child Ought to Know*, he argued that parents were the individuals who were "best fitted . . . to create in the child the ability to interpret speech by means of the eye, and the habit of expecting to get ideas by watching the face of the speaker" (p. xiv). The parent-centered and individualized instruction that Wright had in mind was to commence before children attended school. He explained that "in the development of the human mind there is a certain period when all conditions are favorable for the acquisition of speech and language" (p. xviii).

Backlash Against Special Educators

Holmes (1915) noted the impressive rate at which special education had been expanding. Like many of his professional colleagues, he pointed to some of the administrative and programmatic problems that were associated with this rapid growth. He paid special attention to the severe shortage of trained teachers. Like Holmes, Goddard (1917) called attention to problems caused by the sudden growth of special education. Goddard agreed with Holmes that the shortage of qualified teachers was a matter about which the public should be concerned. However, Goddard observed other problems that were disquieting. Some of these problems had resulted from school administrators who had assigned a high priority to the creation of special education programs. Although this priority had been applauded by some educational constituencies, it had been resented by others. Those school administrators and teachers who were not involved in special education had been irritated. Parents with children in regular education programs also had been disgruntled.

Goddard (1917) gave specific examples of accusations that malcontents had made about special education. For example, they had charged that "the child who can [learn], the normal child, is being neglected" (p. 1). In fact, they had alleged that "so much attention has been paid of late to . . . stupid [*sic*] children . . . that citizens and even educators are complaining" (p. 1). Some of the critics were upset by the immense publicity that the special educators had been able to create. These critics believed that this publicity had been generated after a group of school administrators had proclaimed "that more unusual methods must be followed if [children with disabilities] were to gain anything from their school activities" (p. 1).

After dutifully restating these criticisms, Goddard attempted to dispute them. For example, he disagreed with the critics who suggested that special educators had generated attention through pedagogical fads. Attempting to be even-handed, Goddard did concede that the special educators had promoted their new field of study effectively. However, he believed that they had created excitement by increasing the public's awareness of infrequently employed but fundamentally sound pedagogical strategies. To emphasize this point, Goddard restated the historical adage that "any one can teach a bright child, but . . . it takes an expert to teach a stupid [*sic*] one" (1917, p. 1).

The pedagogical practices that special educators were employing had produced a great deal of professional interest. Their research also elicited sizeable public interest. In a preface that she wrote originally in 1916, Bronner (1923) commented on the steady growth of the public interest. Although she was gratified at the enthusiasm, Bronner judged that some it had been undeserved. For example, she was distressed at the popularity of those special educators who had focused a large portion of their research on "individuals of general low intelligence." She recommended that they shift their attention to persons with the "narrower types of defect" (p. v). Irrespective of the types of learners on whom special educational researchers had focused, Anderson (1917) had been skeptical about using their studies to justify scholastic activities. He lectured his professional colleagues that "the work for defectives in the public schools is so new and experimental" that it should be "verified or discarded as later developments prove them right or wrong" (p. v).

Nash and Porteus (1919) agreed with Anderson (1917) that the research about special learning was too new to be trusted. They cautioned that "the problem of the right educational treatment of defectives has met with only partial solution" (p. 1). Nash and Porteus were suspicious of studies in which the researchers had examined special educational techniques but failed to observe the impact of those techniques on students in actual school settings. In fact, Nash and Porteus even questioned many of the studies in which the researchers had engaged students in their classes. They explained that the designated classes "are not very special, the children are not properly observed, and no real opportunity is afforded them" (p. v).

Summary

During the nineteenth century, persons with disabilities had been sequestered in asylums, special hospitals, prisons, or reformatories. Even many of the citizens who supported these facilities recognized their drawbacks. Restrictive facilities were expensive to build and operate. They comprised deplorable living quarters. They were too crowded to accommodate additional inmates.

Members of the public searched for alternatives. They began to send disabled adults to experimental facilities at which they could farm, assist with institutional chores, or work in neighboring factories. These new facilities had several humanitarian advantages, including opportunities to improve the quality of patients' lives. They also had practical benefits, such as the capacity to accommodate additional patients and operate for relatively modest costs.

As for children with disabilities, most of them were assigned to the public schools. Although school-based care did not require the construction of new buildings, it did necessitate the hiring of trained staffs. Realizing that few of their current teachers were prepared to instruct disabled youths, school administrators collaborated with professors to develop specialized coursework and innovative internships.

3

Distinctive Pedagogy

In America, different state legislatures . . . made a favourable [sic] report on the results of training idiots [sic], which . . . cannot be regarded as so much empty compliment, since it was followed by a grant of public money.

—*Ireland, 1877*

At the beginning of the twentieth century, reformers raised humanitarian, legal, and fiscal objections to the ways in which disabled persons were being treated. The alternative treatments that they recommended for adults included community-based programs. School-based programs were some of the alternatives that they recommended for children. They urged that the staffs of these new programs employ extraordinary pedagogical techniques, such as those that European educators already had implemented.

Early European Efforts to Teach Children With Disabilities

Nineteenth-century European educators had been able to arrange clean and comfortable facilities for persons with disabilities. They had been able to introduce humane types of care. They even had created educational opportunities for persons with disabilities. As they were implementing their visionary initiatives, the Europeans educators advised their American colleagues about their progress.

With regard to their progress in establishing educational opportunities for persons with disabilities, the Europeans provided the Americans with several prototypes. For example, they had established schools that were intended exclusively for blind children (Winzer, 1993). They also had organized schools for deaf children

(Winzer, 1993). The Europeans even had educated children with severe mental disabilities. In an early report entitled *Schools in Lunatic Asylums*, Brigham (1845) confirmed that "the education of the insane, [*sic*] has been attempted in some Asylums [*sic*]" (p. 284). Brigham added that the instructors in the asylum-based programs had achieved "considerable success."

Brigham (1845) admired those persons who had organized special schools within asylums. He was convinced that these schools had a positive impact on patients. Brigham reported that the lives of asylum residents had been transformed after their "faculties which have been long dormant have been roused, the memory improved, fresh objects of interest created for fixing the wandering mind, and luring it away from distempered fancies" (p. 285). Brigham predicted that "the time is not far distant when [schools for persons with disabilities] will be common in all Institutions [*sic*] for the cure of the Insane [*sic*], and be considered as among the most important of remedial measures" (p. 284).

Writing originally in 1858, Bucknill and Tuke (1968) had published a book with a cumbersome title: *A Manual of Psychological Medicine—Containing the History, Nosology, Description, Statistics, Diagnosis, Pathology, and Treatment of Insanity*. In this classic text, the authors revealed some of the sophisticated insights that nineteenth-century European educators had formed and the progressive practices that they had initiated. Bucknill and Tuke indicated that "in asylum management we find school classes, periodical publications, and a lending library, of great importance in affording relief to the monotony of confinement" (pp. 499–500). The two scholars referred to one British institution in which an experienced schoolmaster had offered evening classes in reading, writing and arithmetic. This schoolmaster had been assisted by some of the attendants at the asylum.

Almost two decades after he had written his text with Bucknill, Daniel Tuke published a study about the educational services at one British asylum. In that later study, Daniel Tuke (1875) reported that 200 of the 1039 inmates at this institution had been attending school. Actually, the asylum contained two schools. One of these was reserved for male patients; a separate school was available to female patients. These schools, which had been operating since 1855, currently employed six teachers. Even though he was an advocate of these schools, Tuke did acknowledge the criticism that some individuals had directed against them. He also provided a retort to this criticism.

> To those who are disposed to be skeptical as to the utility of asylum schools, who think that after all they are somewhat of a pretence and a show, I would ask—Is it likely that the governors of the Richmond Asylum would be willing to spend upwards of £580 a year upon them in remunerating their teachers, unless the

results prove their undeniable utility? Or is it probable, that if it be a delusion, an experiment tried in 1855 should have resulted in a [*sic*] asylum which shows such unmistakable signs of vitality in 1875? (p. 3)

Daniel Tuke (1875) had made the preceding remarks about the school at the Richmond Asylum. He provided only sketchy information about the type of instruction and curriculum to which the Richmond Asylum students had been exposed. Tuke was similarly vague about the benefits of the scholastic activities. However, he did comment on the learners' positive emotional responses to that instruction. Daniel Tuke recounted that "I asked several [patients] whether they enjoyed these lessons, and they assured me they did" (p. 2). He added that "there was a great difference in the expression of those who were being taught, [*sic*] and in their responsiveness to the questions put to them" (p. 2).

Although he did not elaborate about the curriculum that was being employed at the Richmond Asylum, Daniel Tuke (1875) felt that it was reflected in the weekly schedules of the 180 females and the 120 males who were involved in academic learning. These schedules are illustrated in Figure 3.1. They revealed that the asylum's instruction was differentiated for learners at three levels of aptitude. The schedules also indicated the general academic competencies that the curriculum comprised. These competencies included reading, writing, arithmetic, grammar, geography, and music.

Daniel Tuke (1875) recommended that all asylum administrators establish schools comparable to that at the Richmond asylum. He explained that "the gloomy monotony which is apt to creep into these institutions would be greatly lessened, if not prevented, by systematic instruction imparted in an able and interesting manner" (p. 7). Daniel Tuke added that classroom-based learning "brings a number of patients together, and subjects them to a certain amount of wholesome rivalry." He concluded that "it seems to me, indeed, impossible that that the occupation and diversion of the mind which a school . . . provides can be other than beneficial" (p. 7).

Édouard Seguin

Most nineteenth-century educators did not see a need to educate students with disabilities in distinctive fashions. Daniel Tuke (1875) was one of the educators in this large group. Tuke had published detailed schedules for the activities of the patients at the Richmond Asylum. A footnote to these documents indicated that the male students at this asylum had been receiving religious and academic instruction. This instance, in which religion was blended with academics, was not an isolated case. Much of the nineteenth-century instruction that was delivered to persons with disabilities was religious. In fact,

TIME TABLE OF RICHMOND ASYLUM MALE NATIONAL SCHOOL.

Morning	JUNIOR DIVISION.	MIDDLE DIVISION.	SENIOR DIVISION.
8.45 to 9	INSPECTION AS TO CLEANLINESS.		
9 to 9½	DESKS.—Writing.	FLOOR.—Reading.	CLASS ROOM.—Principles of Arithmetic.
9½ to 10	FLOOR.—Reading and Explanation or Arithmetic.	CLASS ROOM.—Geography and Object Lesson alternately.	DESKS.—Writing and Drawing alternately.
10 to 10½	VOCAL AND INSTRUMENTAL MUSIC.		
10½ to 11½	RECREATION AND OUT-DOOR AMUSEMENTS.		
11½ to 12	CLASS ROOM.—Object Lesson.	DESKS.—Writing and Dictation alternately.	FLOOR.—Reading and Grammar on alternate days.
12 to 12½	DESKS.—Arithmetic.	FLOOR.—Arithmetic.	CLASS ROOM.—Object Lesson and Geography, alternately.
Evening, 3 to 4	MIXED CONCERT CLASS ON WEDNESDAYS AND FRIDAYS.		
6½ to 7½	READINGS.—Object Lesson: Geography.	GEOGRAPHY.—Descriptive and Physical —Reading from different authors.	READINGS.—With Explanation.

NOTE.—Religious Instruction is given on Fridays, from 11½ until 12½ o'clock; the ordinary school business begins an hour earlier during the summer than in the winter half-year.

RICHMOND ASYLUM FEMALE NATIONAL SCHOOL.

	OCCUPATION OF SCHOOL TIME.		
Morning Time	JUNIOR DIVISION.	MIDDLE DIVISION.	SENIOR DIVISION.
9.45 to 10	INSPECTION OF PUPILS.		
10 to 10½	Reading and Spelling.	Arithmetic.	Writing and Dictation.
10½ to 11	Marching to Music.	Reading and Spelling.	Arithmetic and Drawing alternately.
11 to 11½	Object Lesson: Mondays, Wednesdays, and Fridays. Tables, counting on Ball-Frame: Tuesdays, Thursdays, and Saturdays.	Writing and Dictation alternately. Geography on Saturdays.	Reading, Spelling, and Explanation. Geography on Saturdays.
11½ to 12½	RECREATION.		
12½ to 1	Writing and marking Figures on Slates.	Geography: Mondays and Wednesdays. Grammar: Tuesdays and Thursdays.	Singing. Geography: Mondays and Wednesdays.
1 to 1½	Singing.	Singing.	Grammar: Tuesdays and Thursdays.
	EVENING SCHOOL.		
7 to 7½	Writing: Mondays, Wednesdays, and Fridays.	Writing: Mondays, Wednesdays, and Fridays.	Writing: Mondays, Wednesdays, and Fridays.
7½ to 8	Singing: Mondays and Wednesdays. Reading: Fridays.	Singing: Mondays and Wednesdays. Reading: Fridays.	Singing: Mondays and Wednesdays. Reading: Fridays.

NOTE.—Mixed Concert Classes on Wednesdays and Fridays, from 3 to 4 o'clock in the afternoon. Separate Religious Instruction, in the respective places of worship, from 12½ to 1½ o'clock on Fridays. Excursion to Park, Zoological and Botanical Gardens in the summer season, on Tuesdays and Fridays.

Figure 3.1. Late Nineteenth-Century Schedule at a British Asylum.

many patients received religious instruction exclusively. In those rare cases in which academic instruction was provided, it was sporadic and disorganized.

Édouard Seguin was one of the first educators to realize that students with disabilities would benefit from a distinctive type of pedagogy. He devised pedagogical techniques that were different from those that had been developed for the students in regular education classrooms. In an early historical account, Walter Fernald (1893) wrote with admiration about the book in which Seguin had expressed this insight. Fernald reported that "in 1846 Dr [*sic*] Seguin published his classical and comprehensive 'Treatise on Idiocy,' [*sic*] which was crowned by the Academy [*sic*] and has continued to be the standard text-book [*sic*] for all interested in the education of idiots up to the present time" (p. 204). Alexander Johnson (1899) also lauded Seguin for his insights about pedagogy. Johnson wrote that Seguin deserved to be called "the apostle of the Idiot" because he had devised an instructional approach that "was plainly indicated as the correct one" (p. 463). Several years later, Norsworthy (1906) joined those scholars who had bestowed accolades upon Seguin. Norsworthy wrote that "it is to Edward Seguin that the honour [*sic*] belongs of having created a real method . . . for the treatment and education of idiots" and that this method was "still followed in general in the education of the feeble-minded" (p. 2).

Goddard (1923), who was one of the preeminent scholars of this era, provided still another testimonial about Seguin's extraordinary impact on special education. In the introduction to one of his textbooks, Goddard wrote that special education emerged in 1837, "when the famous Dr. Seguin began his work in systematic training of school children" (1923, p. xix). In an earlier report, Goddard (1912) had written about Seguin in an extremely effusive manner. Goddard noted that "under the inspiration of the immortal Seguin it was discovered much could be done" for persons with disabilities. However, Goddard lamented that some of Seguin's disciples had taken their master's concepts to extremes. He wrote that these followers had become so zealous that they had begun to proclaim that persons with disabilities "could even be cured" (1912, p. 119).

In his own writings, Seguin eloquently represented his views about pedagogy. In fact, the clarity with which Seguin conveyed his insights was partially responsible for his enviable reputation. Seguin's eloquence was evident in many of his books, including a work that he had published originally in 1866. In that book, Seguin (1907) had noted that persons with disabilities had "been educated in all times by the devotion of kind-hearted and intelligent persons" (p. 9). Seguin then pointed out that the individuals who had delivered this care had employed "the best means they could borrow from ordinary schools" (p. 9). Seguin had a different instructional approach in mind. As an alternative to transposing techniques that had been developed for regular education classrooms, he wished to create a distinctive pedagogy.

Seguin (1907) wrote persuasively about the novel pedagogy that he envisaged. For example, he adjured teachers that "two successive lessons shall not employ the same set of organs, nor, exact the use of the same intellectual functions" (p. 192). Seguin thought that systematic changes in modes of learning and methods of instruction could reduce "the oral fatigue which results from protracted and often unsuccessful contacts of obedience and understanding" (p. 192).

Seguin provided numerous additional recommendations about ways to instruct children with disabilities. Some of his suggestions were so effective that instructors followed them for decades. For example, Seguin had insisted that special educators should methodically maintain records about their students.

> It is yet [the teacher's] duty to note anything particular which has transpired about the children, or any remarks of hers upon the teaching, suggested by her own experience of the day. These notes cannot be confided to fugacious memory, but must be written in a durable form and laid like the material for the foundation of a better edifice than the present method is, after having been discussed in teachers' meetings, and submitted to the repeated tests of experience. (1907, p. 192)

Writing in the early 1920s, Shuttleworth and Potts (1922) illustrated several learning devices that had been designed by Seguin in the middle of the preceding century but that were still popular. Two of these devices, the size board and the form board, are illustrated in Figure 3.2. Shuttleworth and Potts explained that both of these learning instruments developed "accuracy not only of grasping movements, but of capacity for adjustment of insets to their appropriate cavities" (p. 216).

Seguin had wished to make special education systematic. Although he attempted to persuade others to adopt his viewpoint, he was only somewhat successful. Duncan (1866) was a British scholar who alluded to the prevailing skepticism about recommendations of the sort that Seguin had been offering. Duncan underscored this point in the preface to a textbook about special education in Great Britain.

> A book on a rational system of education of the "feeble-minded," imbecile and idiotic, has long been required. It is well known that but a few of the unfortunate beings, for whose benefit such a work might be written, ever have the advantage of a carefully adapted training; and that the majority suffer both from unreasonable as well as from inefficient treatment. (p. vii)

Duncan (1866) had believed that Seguin's work had changed the attitudes of many of the British physicians and educators who were providing care to disabled persons. To substantiate this point, he reproduced a section of a current British report. In that report, the authors had noted that "the benefits to be derived . . . from a distinctive system [of special education], and from persevering endeavors to develope [*sic*] the dormant powers, physical and intellectual, are now so fully established, that any argument upon the subject would be superfluous" (passage from the *Report of Lunacy Commissioners*, 1865, as quoted by Duncan, 1866, p. 189).

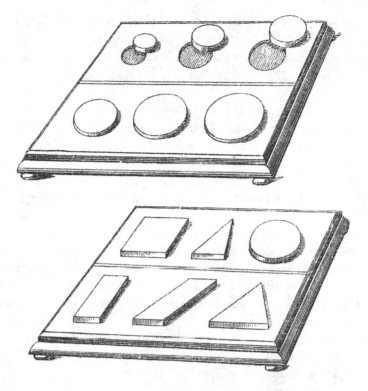

Figure 3.2. Nineteenth-Century Devices Adapted for Special Education Classrooms.

Tredgold (1908) was a British scholar who wrote a popular book about persons with disabilities. In that book, he agreed with Seguin's fundamental assumptions. For example, Tredgold judged that special learners would benefit from distinctive and systematic types of instruction. Like Seguin, he urged that "school training" involve methods that were "more systematized" than those typically used in private schools or philanthropic institutions. Furthermore, Tredgold endorsed a comprehensive approach to school-based training in which students would develop their sensory skills, refine their motor patterns, learn about morality, and master "intellectual" objectives.

William Ireland

Although one cannot confirm the precise degree to which nineteenth-century instructors were aware of specialized pedagogy, it is clear that some of them were not only aware but also employing it. Ireland (1877) wrote one of the first reports about the distinctive pedagogies that could benefit special learners. In this book, Ireland quoted a passage in which one of his contemporaries gave sophisticated advice about the way to set educational goals for students with severe disabilities.

> The measure of good effected [*sic*] . . . depends upon "the distance which sepa-rated the starting-point from that reached." To teach an idiot, who, to begin with, cannot walk, crams his food into his mouth with his hands, and bolts it, using his teeth mainly to bite viciously any one [*sic*] who comes near him; who never puts on clothes or takes them off except by tearing them; who has no more cleanliness and decency in his natural habits than an animal living in the fields, and incomparably less, therefore, than a dog or a cat, which respects the cleanli-ness of the house; to teach such an idiot to walk, to work, and to play, to dig with a spade, or to kick a football, to feed himself with a knife and a fork, to dress and undress himself, to wash, and behave in a cleanly and decent manner, to kiss his com-panion instead of biting him, to have the use even of a few words which he articu-lates and understands, even if he should not be able to read well, or to write a fair copy—I say that the difference between the starting-point and the winning-post, to me seems greater in such a case than when a weak-minded man learns to build the model of a ship. (John Charles Bucknill, Lord Chancellor's Visitor of Lunatics, 1873, as quoted by Ireland, 1877, pp. 329–330)

Ireland (1877) provided anecdotal information about the idiosyncratic pedagogy that some instructors were employing to teach reading. For example, he described instructors who had "resorted to the device of tracing letters in phosphoric acid on the wall of a dark room, in order to rouse the languid attention of the child" (p. 318). Ireland assumed that the eccentricity of the preceding approach would be apparent to his readers. Nonetheless, he adjured them to consider using it and a full range of other options. He pointed out that teachers would need these options in order to teach students to read in English. He reassured them that learning to read in English was extremely complicated because the language contained so many phonetic irregular-ities. At the same time that he was advising them about ways to develop reading skills, Ireland reassured teachers that they should not worry excessively about those children who did not become readers. He counseled them that illiterate students still could "be educated in a great variety of ways" (p. 318).

Ireland (1877) believed that persons with disabilities could master some arith-metic skills. He thought that these skills were "necessary for so many transactions of life" (p. 317). Even though he realized that special mathematical instruction required teachers to exhibit "more than usual patience," he counseled them that their efforts would be worthwhile. Furthermore, they could simplify their instruction by building on the interests and dispositions that their children already exhibited. Ireland pointed out that "the abstract idea of quantity, represented by expressions, such as many, big, plenty, are generally taken up spontaneously" and that "most children who are educable at all can distinguish between a big bit of bread and a small one, or a cup of milk full or half full" (pp. 317–318).

Ireland (1877) provided teachers with detailed information about the pedagogy that they could use to help children understand mathematical concepts. This pedagogy paired mathematical learning with the manipulation of tangible items.

> [Students] should be carefully exercised in counting objects, reckoning money, the number of days in the week and hours in the day. . . . Numbers with them must always be taught upon the object—upon the bead-frame, for example, or to count a certain number of beads or pebbles; anything will do if it be movable, and all of the same kind. See that the child can set apart so many beads, or string so many beads on a wire, and then teach him to repeat the corresponding number. When he can count thirty the pupil may commence simple addition—that is, by adding twos and threes together upon the ball-frame. About the same time they begin to learn the written symbols of figures, but it will be long before these can be substituted for the actual numbers counted out. (p. 317)

Ireland (1877) was particularly impressed with an Italian educator who had devised a special instructional technique. This educator had matched numerals with arrays of dots. The arrays depicted the values of the numerals. Figure 3.3, which is an illustration from Ireland's book (p. 317), demonstrated one of the ways in which this technique could be used for instruction.

Ireland (1877) also gave advice about writing instruction. In this advice, which was as insightful as that which he had given about reading and mathematics instruction, he emphasized the importance of carefully assessing the results of instruction. He warned teachers who ignored his advice that they would lead students awry. Ireland gave the example of students with disabilities who had learned "to trace letters without being able to read them" (p. 322). He added quickly that "some boys of considerable intelligence are very bad writers" (p. 322). Despite these cautionary notes, Ireland was enthusiastic about writing instruction. He carefully described practical exercises to simplify the instruction. For example, he advised the teachers to allow their students to write "on a slate, after which they may be taught to write over a traced copy" (p. 322). A strong proponent of both patience and persistence, Ireland noted that "sometimes the hand of the pupil requires to be guided by the teacher for weeks, or even months, before he can form a letter" (p. 322).

Given the inordinate amount of attention that special learners required, some wealthy parents had hired private governesses to instruct their children. Even

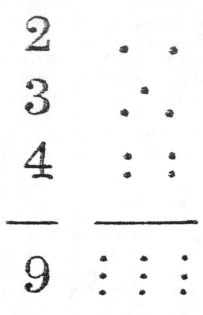

Figure 3.3. A Nineteenth-Century Learning Activity Adapted for Special Education Classrooms.

though this practice had superficial attractions, Ireland (1877) was not enthusiastic about it. He wrote bluntly that "I do not remember ever to have heard of much being done in this way" (p. 297). Ireland explained that the average governess "lacks the conviction, derived from experience or observation, that her efforts will not be thrown away, and the tact acquired by practice of getting round, past, or under difficulties" (p. 297).

Later Nineteenth-Century European Pedagogues

Ireland had predicted that the book he had published in 1877 would be read by physicians. However, he had hoped that it also would be read by guardians, caregivers, philanthropists, and the many members of the public who were concerned about persons with disabilities. Morgan (1896), who also hoped to attract a broad range of readers, published a report about "word blindness" in the *British Medical Journal*. Morgan recounted a case study of a young man who, in spite of "laborious and persistent training," could "only spell out words of one syllable" (p. 1378). He pointed out that this behavior "follows upon no injury but, but is evidently congenital" (p. 1378). Morgan's fascination with this particular student intensified after he learned that "the schoolmaster who has taught him for some years says that he would be the smartest lad in the school if the instruction were entirely oral" (p. 1378).

Although he was interested primarily in the physiological etiology of word blindness, Morgan (1896) carefully described the pedagogical antidotes that teachers had employed. Morgan focused his attention on the teachers who had corrected one student's case of "letter blindness." These teachers corrected a case of "word blindness" that the same student later developed. The successful teachers had relied on the systematic and "constant application" of academic activities. Since these teachers were still tutoring the young man at the time that Morgan was writing, Morgan speculated that "it will be interesting to see what effect further training will have" (p. 1378).

Hinshelwood (1900) was another scholar who was concerned about word blindness. Although he had investigated only several cases, Hinshelwood was convinced that word blindness was a common disability. He also was convinced that word blindness required a special type of pedagogy.

> Although I have not been able to bring forward more than these four cases as illustrations of this congenital form of "word-blindness" I have but little doubt that these are by no means so rare as the absence of recorded cases would lead us to infer. Their rarity is, I think, accounted for by the fact that when they do occur they are not recognized. It is a matter of the highest importance to recognize the cause and the true nature of this difficulty in learning to read which is experienced by these children, otherwise they may be harshly treated as imbeciles or incorrigibles and either neglected or flogged for a defect for which they are in no wise responsible. The recognition of the true character of the difficulty will lead the parents and teachers of these children . . . to overcome the difficulty by patient and persistent training. (p. 1508)

In addition to calling attention to novel types of disabilities, late nineteenth-century researchers and practitioners singled out some of the instructional interventions in which they had confidence. For example, Hinshelwood (1917) reminisced about the success that early researchers and educators had with the "old-fashioned" phonics approach. He explained, that "the child has simply to recognize by sight the individual letters, and can now read words by spelling them aloud, and thus appealing to its [*sic*] auditory memory" (p. 107). Hinshelwood added that phonics-based instruction was especially well-suited to "the child with defective visual and good auditory memory" because that child would have "the visual impressions of the words deepened and strengthened by the constant associationship [*sic*] with the impressions already made in its [*sic*] auditory centre [*sic*]" (p. 107).

Early American Efforts to Teach Children With Disabilities

A group of American reformers wished to help persons with disabilities. In many ways, they followed the pattern of the Europeans. Walter Fernald (1893; 1917), who was American, had referred to the peculiar influence of early nineteenth-century European initiatives on American education. Fernald observed that "the published description of the methods and results of these European schools attracted much interest and attention in America" (1917, p. 35). Daniel Tuke (1892a), who was British, later made this same point. Tuke noted that "the movements for the betterment of those deranged in mind, in the various countries of Europe, as also in the United Sates, will show the march of events to have been in the same direction, although as a matter of fact in very different degrees" (p. 26).

Daniel Tuke had concluded that the North American initiatives lagged significantly behind those in Europe. Like Tuke, Arlidge (1859) was British. However, Arlidge may have been the only British scholar who judged that the Americans had made greater progress than the Europeans. Arlidge complimented the Americans on several counts. For example, he believed they were to be commended because their "public asylums are not branded with the appellation 'pauper,' they are called 'State Asylums,' and every facility is offered for the admission of cases . . . whatever their previous civil condition" (p. 28). Arlidge added that "there is not in the United States the feeling of false pride, of imaginary family dishonour [*sic*] or discredit, to the same extent which is observed in this country, when it pleases Providence [*sic*] to visit a relative with mental derangement,—[*sic*] to oppose the transmission to a place of treatment" (p. 28).

Ireland (1898) was another British scholar who detected growing excitement about special education in the United States. In the preface to one of his books, Ireland (1898) commented on this trend. He indicated that he was encouraged because the members of "the rising school of psychology in the United States" had shown an interest in his own research. He then contrasted the situation in America with that in England. Ireland felt that the "students of psychology in Great Britain" had not given sufficient respect to his research. Although he had made it clear that his feelings had been hurt, Ireland had not despaired "of receiving some little attention" from the British group.

Most scholars did not share Arlidge's and Ireland's flattering appraisal of the progress that the North Americans had made. Although he conceded that some Americans and Canadians had attempted to replicate the British programs, Daniel Tuke (1885) questioned the degree to which they had been successful. Having visited some of the North

American facilities, Tuke was in a position to make this challenge. On the basis of observations that he had made during that tour, he concluded that "it is a cause of regret that the condition in which [the author] found certain asylums in Canada left him no alternative, consistent with the truth, but to paint them in the colours [*sic*] which presented themselves to his view" (p. ii). Tuke was similarly distraught by the conditions that he had witnessed in the asylums of the United States.

Like Daniel Tuke, Seguin (1870) and Ireland (1877) had made journeys to North America to tour special educational facilities. Each of these scholars wrote precise reports about the instructional practices that they had observed. Although they found some positive developments, both Seguin and Ireland were struck by how recently those changes had occurred. Seguin (1870) noted that "a little more than twenty years ago, there was no educational establishment for idiots in the United States" (p. 10). However, Seguin added that by 1870 there were "at least nine in all, where above one thousand children are under instruction" (p. 10). Ireland (1877) later agreed with Seguin. A table (Figure 3.4) in Ireland's book identified the few American schools in which the staffs had attempted to provide special educational services.

Some of the teachers in American institutions did not set their instructional expectations as high as their European counterparts had done. As an example, Wilbur (1862), who described himself as an American teacher "devoted to a class known as idiots," did not maintain a high regard of his students.

> Viewed as subjects of education, we may speak of the class as incapable of sustaining ordinary social relations, and as insusceptible of development, by the ordinary methods of instruction. In other words, the problem of education in the case of idiots is complicated by the inertia or inactivity of the in-dwelling sprit; by the imperfect means of communication with it [*sic*] from without; by the weakness or deficiency of the mental faculties; by the limited number and feebleness of the incentives and motives that can be brought to bear upon it [*sic*]; by the absence or impotence of the moral sense, and finally, by the physiological limitation to the development process in each individual case. (p. 8)

Many American educators shared Wilbur's dismal view of special learners.

Changing American Attitudes Toward Special Instruction

Historically, the public's attitudes toward persons with disabilities had been negative. However, American educators and scholars were encouraged by the changes that they observed at the end of the nineteenth century and the beginning of the twentieth century. In addition to detecting changes, they thought that they detected a predictable

UNITED STATES.

	Founded.	Number of Pupils.	How Supported.
Barre, Massachusetts .	1848	70	{ Private institution.
Boston, do. .	1848	80	State.
Syracuse, New York .	1851	215	State.
Media, Pennsylvania .	1853	225	State.
Lakeville, Connecticut } .	1858	85	State.
Columbus, Ohio .	1857	408	State.
Frankfort, Kentucky .	1860	120	State.
New York City, Randall's Island } .	1860	183	City.
Jacksonville, Illinois .	1865	100	State.
Fayville, Massachusetts } .	1870	12	Private.
Glenwood, Iowa . .	1876	14	State.

Figure 3.4. An 1877 List of the American Schools with Special Education Programs.

pattern to them. For example, they believed that initially only the most progressive members of the public had been receptive to special education. Walter Fernald (1917) commented on this trend. After he had reviewed the nineteenth-century initiatives to educate persons with disabilities, he wrote that these early efforts "were practically all begun as tentative experiments in the face of great public distrust and doubt as to the value of the results" (p. 39). After these experiments were demonstrated to be effective, the general public became more supportive.

Barr (1904), who was a physician at the Pennsylvania Training School for Feeble-minded Children, also commented on the pattern that had characterized the public's changing attitudes. In an early history of special education, he acknowledged that the general public was skeptical about the value of special education. In fact, Barr professed his own continuing conviction about "the utter hopelessness of cure, and also the needless waste of energy in attempting to teach an idiot" (p. vii). The only positive prospect that Barr ascribed to special education was the possibility that it could prevent children with disabilities from degenerating to lower levels of immorality.

Before they could implement special education programs in the public schools, the advocates of the programs had to convince reluctant school administrators that special education had value. However, those school administrators who were persuaded faced problems significant problems of their own. For example, they had to deal with the teachers who refused to adapt the traditional curriculum for the students with disabilities who were admitted to their schools. Because problems of this sort were pervasive, Wallin (1914) suspected that the individual needs of many special learners were being ignored. To make this point, he identified 14 American cities in which special education classes had been organized from 1896 to 1906. Although he commended the communities for these initiatives, Wallin questioned the instruction that they had been offering. He wrote that "although these classes undoubtedly contained seriously backward or feeble-minded children, it is not apparent that the program of studies consisted of special class work" (p. 389).

Many Americans assumed that the fates of all children with disabilities were hopeless. Although reform-minded educators disagreed, they disagreed cautiously. Barnes (1908) was a professor who argued that "defective children" fell into "many classes" and needed "widely different treatment" (p. 1121). This type of logic began to strike more and more persons as reasonable. While they were considering the new arguments in favor of special education, American citizens simultaneously were learning about the progressive, student-centered models of education that the Europeans had implemented. The Americans learned from professors such as Doll (1919), who testified about America's great indebtedness to the French system of education. Doll thought that this indebtedness was "particularly true with regard to the study of feeble-mindedness" (p. 187). As an increasing numbers of parents discovered the European viewpoints, they placed pressure on school administrators and teachers to change their parochial views. They demanded that they replicate the European models of instruction.

Findlay (1911) was another educator who called attention to the ways in which the attitudes toward learners with disabilities were changing. Findlay specifically castigated tradition-dominated teachers who had ignored current psychological research and retained archaic assumptions about genetic determinism. He advised these teachers that "public opinion has rejected the pedantry of narrow scholarship imposed on children in days gone by" (p. 27). Findlay admonished them to surrender their "hold upon the curriculum of the school" (p. 27).

Farrell (1914d), who was the administrator in charge of special education for New York City's public schools, became a popular and eloquent spokesperson for the new perspective on special learning. Her logical acumen, scholarship, and rhetorical skills were evident in the way that she explained some of the pedagogical changes that were transpiring in the schools.

> The problem of backwardness in children is one which necessarily occupies the attention of school administrators. A solution was expected by many when medical inspection of school children became general. Undertaken first as a public health measure, the medical inspection was soon centred [*sic*] on the detection and the correction of physical defects found in school children. . . . [Although] teachers

and school superintendents looked for the almost total elimination of the problem of retardation when physical defects were corrected . . . this . . . was not the
case. Certain children were still unable to make progress. Discipline was no whit
easier. Another remedy was needed. (pp. iii–iv)

In an earlier report, Farrell (1908b) had written that educators had failed to
develop the distinctive pedagogies that special learners required. She gave two examples to substantiate this point.

We do not have any new methods for teaching reading: we use a combination of all
good methods, sentence, word and phonic; we have no new device for developing
the sense of quantity or of quality: we weigh [*sic*] measure, compare, reckon; we have
only such means as are open to all for the training of childhood. (pp. 1134–1135)

Because they had not developed distinctive pedagogies, special educators frequently relied on general philosophical principles to guide the ways in which they
instructed children with disabilities. Farrell (1908b) described two of these principles.

The general principle upon which all education of mentally defective children is based
is: "Begin where the defect or disease impeded the normal development." This point
may be determined in either of two ways: the teacher may begin with those exercises
which naturally a boy of given years should be able to do, and from that work backward to the point where the child can accomplish a given exercise. . . . The opposite
process is that which begins with the most elementary workings of the child's neuro-
muscular system, and climbs upward by means of very short, definite, more complex workings until the arrest in development has been reached. (p. 1132)

Farrell referred to approaches that followed the initial philosophical principle as
"negative procedures." She referred to approaches that followed the second principle as "positive procedures." As her readers must have anticipated, she endorsed
the positive procedures.

Farrell had called attention to the changing American attitudes toward the disabled children who were being sent to the schools. Merrill (1918), who was a research
assistant at the Minnesota School for the Feeble-Minded, also called attention to the
shifting attitudes. After reviewing the school-attendance laws that had been implemented during the late nineteenth and early twentieth centuries, she indicated that
the newer state regulations had spurred alternative models of instruction.

Since universal compulsory education has placed in the public schools children
of widely varying abilities, within the last twenty-five years the schools have
made special efforts to replace the old procrustean effort to adjust the child to the

school with the more humane modern methods. . . . The special or ungraded class in the public schools usually includes at least two types of children, the temporarily backward and the feeble-minded. Its objects are two: to relieve the regular grades and to educate or train the atypical child. (p. 90)

Merrill (1918) added several additional observations that had political overtones. For example, she thought that discussions about the new models of instruction had confused the public. Inaccurate information, which had been endemic to these discussions, had been one of the primary reasons for the confusion. Merrill accused overzealous supporters of misrepresenting the actual degree to which the new instructional models had been implemented in the schools. To prove this point, Merrill referred to the special education programs in Cleveland, Ohio. The students in these programs had been sorted into two groups, those who were "socially competent" and those who were "socially incompetent." Depending on the category into which they had been placed, the students should have received a distinctive type of instruction. However, Merrill admitted that all of Cleveland's special learners were being taught as if they were socially incompetent. This expedient procedure was being followed because classes for socially incompetent students were "usually the only special classes in the school" (p. 89).

Late Nineteenth-Century American Pedagogy

Late nineteenth-century researchers and educators described some of the novel approaches that were becoming available to students with disabilities. Scott (1899) made extremely detailed remarks about a program at the "vacation school for the feeble-minded." As an indication of the specificity of her remarks, she indicated that the program in question had been started by the Chicago Woman's Club, located at 4634 Ashland Avenue, and funded with an annual budget of $75.00. Scott lauded the program as the "first day school [sic] work of the kind ever attempted in this country" (p. 65). However, Scott did add parenthetically that the Chicago program had been modeled on programs in England, "where the education and welfare of this class of children is receiving wide attention" (p. 65). Norsworthy (1906), who was a professor of educational psychology at Teachers College, agreed with Scott's last point. He also judged that "in America, attention was attracted to this new field of work [with persons with disabilities] by the interest shown abroad" (p. 3).

Even though most turn-of-the century observers conceded that special education was more advanced in England than it was in the United States, they recognized that several American programs had been initiated during the 1800s. Barnes (1908) reported that "since 1890 we have been slowly establishing in all parts of Europe and America special schools for peculiar children in connection with the public schools of the municipalities or states" (p. 1118). Despite this guardedly optimistic assessment, Barnes acknowledged that "in country districts we must still get along as best we can, by removing the more difficult children to residential homes" (p. 1123).

Arthur Holmes (1912) reminisced about some of the nineteenth-century American initiatives in special education. For example, he reported about asylum administrators who had opened an experimental state-supported school in New York. Holmes added that one of their primary motives had been to "demonstrate [the experimental school's] value to the law-makers" (p. 24). This facility was so successful that the state legislators eventually provided a permanent budget for it.

Arthur Holmes (1912) also referred to some of the important incidents that had transpired in American schools. He focused on events in Providence, Rhode Island. He cited a report that singled out Providence as "the first city to plan for a complete organization of [special education] classes directly under the city superintendent" (passage from Bulletin No. 14, United States Bureau of Education, 1911, quoted by Holmes, 1912, p. 24). The authors of this Bureau of Education report added that the Providence initiative had involved "six classes for truants and disciplinary cases in 1893, and a separate class for backward children in 1896" (passage from Bulletin No. 14, United States Bureau of Education, 1911, quoted by Holmes, 1912, p. 24). Opposite the page on which he had provided the preceding citation, Holmes placed a contemporary photograph that revealed the changing character of special education. It depicted a public-school classroom in which special learners were being taught living skills. The title indicated that the photographed group comprised "atypical pre-adolescent children at dinner" (Holmes, 1912, p. 27).

Arthur Holmes had called attention to the special education classes that had been established in Providence, Rhode Island. Other educators alluded to the pioneering initiatives in other cities. For example, Lincoln (1903) recounted that the superintendent of Boston "engaged a teacher in the fall of 1898 and placed her over a class of fifteen children in January, 1899" (p. 84). Lincoln added that six additional special education classes were established in Boston during the subsequent six years.

Despite some visionary efforts, special education in the United States continued to trail its British counterpart. One of the reasons for this delay may have been the regressive social attitudes. Consider the reactions of some Rhode Island citizens to the revolutionary work in their community.

> A special class was started in Providence several years ago, the first special class
> in this country. The work there was very severely criticized because one leading

newspaper had published a cartoon labeled, "The Fool Class." Naturally all parents objected to sending their children to the Fool Class. (Johnstone, 1909a, p. 122)

Johnstone (1909a), who had written the preceding passage, believed that school-board members and school administrators did not deserve the credit for the expansion of special educational programs. To the contrary, he estimated that "New York, Boston, Philadelphia, and a half-a-dozen other cities soon had special classes in their schools because the pressure brought to bear was so great that the school board and superintendents could not withstand it" (p. 122).

Shuttleworth (1899) was another scholar who offered data that underscored the differences between the special education programs in Europe and those in the United States. He had genuine reservations about the European initiatives, which he thought had failed to meet the needs of many children. Shuttleworth observed that "in England and Wales about 42,000 children, or one per cent of the elementary school class, between the ages of seven and thirteen . . . are too mentally weak to be taught in ordinary schools, but . . . are neither idiots nor imbeciles" (p. 58). Shuttleworth wanted educational services to be accessible to all of these children. To illustrate how the expansion of services might occur, he summarized the recommendations of a recently convened British committee. This committee specifically had urged increased and improved services for children who were visually impaired or deaf.

[The members of the committee recommend:]

1. That towns with a populations of 10,000 or upwards should establish a special class, or classes, for feebleminded children.
2. That school authorities should have power to provide maintenance in homes or conveyance to and from school when necessary.
3. That school authorities should have power to raise the age for compulsory attendance, when desirable, to sixteen for feebleminded children.
4. That admission to special classes should be made after examination by a medical authority. (Passage from the 1896 report of an ad hoc committee that had been appointed by the Lord President of England's Council on Education, as quoted by Shuttleworth, 1899, p. 59)

Educational reform in the United States lagged behind that in Great Britain. The reluctance of state legislators to enact compulsory school-attendance laws provided an indication of this lag. Not until 1918 had all of the state legislatures established compulsory school-attendance laws. Even after this date, many legislatures exempted children with disabilities from those legal provisions (Yell, Rogers, & Rogers, 1998). As for special education, its scope was less comprehensive in the United States than it was in Great Britain. The type of instruction that special educators provided in the two systems was still another indication of differential progress. Most early twentieth-century educators could discern the gap between the sophisticated pedagogy that had been introduced in Great Britain (Ireland, 1877) and the primitive pedagogy that was being employed in Boston two decades later (Lincoln, 1903). After reviewing Boston's special education programs, Lincoln (1903) commented on its disorganization. He wrote that "there was no requirement, scarcely even a suggestion, as to the results to be sought, or the methods to be used" (p. 84).

Educators in Great Britain had developed systematic identification procedures to determine which students could attend special education classes. Identification of special learners was another academic area in which American educators trailed their British colleagues. Lincoln (1903) chronicled the disorganized way in which Boston educators had been selecting the students for that city's special education programs.

> Previous to the appointment of the first [special education] teacher . . . the names of two hundred pupils had been secured from the masters of schools as unsuited for being taught in the regular classes. From these, after examination, she picked out fifteen of the most urgent cases and became their teacher. Other classes were formed at intervals; and, about three years later, a second inquiry elicited a new series of cases, of which about two hundred have been carefully studied by . . . an unpaid volunteer. (p. 84)

Needless to say, this type of informal screening created variability among the learners who were admitted into special education programs. To illustrate the wide range of the learners that had been admitted into Boston's special education classes, Lincoln (1903) described the 15 students who had been grouped into a single classroom. Lincoln recounted that two of these students "had rickets, six convulsions, one epilepsy, three were seriously deaf, four had difficulty with ordinary movements of walking and skipping, ten spoke with defective articulation, two had deformed palates and only three had good teeth" (pp. 84–85).

Writing at the same time as Lincoln (1903), Chace (1903) also was struck by the range of the disabilities that the children in American special education programs exhibited. She contrasted the American and the German admission procedures. Whereas the American school administrators lacked firm guidelines about the children who were eligible for special education, their German counterparts reserved special classes "solely for the education of mentally deficient children" (p. 386). Chace applauded the Germans for the way in which they had diverted students with disabilities into highly specialized programs. For example, they had separated students with mental disabilities from "the blind and the deaf, those with moral perversion, those backward on account of irregular attendance or illness, those backward in some particular subject, the idiots and the epileptics" (p. 386).

In his reminiscence about American special education, Doll (1928) later made a point similar to that which Chace (1903) had offered. Doll had difficulty drawing conclusions about the effectiveness of the early American special education classrooms. Struck by the variability in the types of students who were assigned to those classes, he attributed this range to the immense discretion that school administrators had employed when admitting students. Doll judged that the school administrators had not been concerned about meeting the needs of students with genuine disabilities so much as they were about ridding their schools of "various sorts of misfits" (p. 145).

Early Twentieth-Century American Pedagogy

American special educators eventually developed a set of tenets to help them teach more effectively. One of these tenets specified that children with disabilities comprised a heterogeneous group. Another tenet specified that children with disabilities required individualized instruction. An increasing number of professional colleagues agreed with these tenets. More and more members of the public agreed with them as well.

Hamilton (1906) was an experienced teacher who supported the use of individualized instruction. She wrote that individualized instruction "reduces the one-sidedness of the pupil, contributes to his symmetry and balance and saves him from the deficiencies of class instruction" (p. 6). Hamilton gave advice to teachers about ways to implement an individualized approach to instruction. For example, she directed them to "recognize individual differences and show the pupil how to study, how to find his errors and correct them and in this way he eventually learns the greater and more important lesson of depending upon himself" (p. 6).

Rosenfeld (1906) had observed instances of individualized instruction while he was touring 16 schools in New York City. He made a detailed report about these instances.

> For drawing and writing less effort is required when the children use large pencils and large scale [*sic*] exercises. They draw and then cut out common objects, such as chair, flag, ladder, and then learn to read and write the name of the object. Often the child is taught to write by having his hand guided by the teacher or some older pupil. The drawings express the child's idea of a given object, as a snowstorm,

park, house, etc., and are crude. Those children who have no ideas of their own are allowed to look at their neighbor's work. (p. 96)

Rosenfeld (1906) also gave specific examples of the ways in which mathematics instruction was being individualized in New York City's special education classrooms.

Individual number work is necessary. Sticks, fingers, shells, beads are used to tell the number story. Some children have no conception of number; [*sic*] can hardly grasp one number a day, and with great difficulty learn them in rotation. Later, playing storekeeper is the subterfuge used to teach the use of the scale, the value of weights and the worth of money. (p. 97)

Groszmann (1907) adjured teachers to refrain from stereotyping "contrary" students. He was worried that the teachers would depict them as individuals with "naturally perverse morality, [*sic*] or at least temporary moral aberration" (p. 93). Groszmann explained that students' contrary behaviors could "be a purely mental symptom, without any moral significance whatever" (p. 93). He encouraged the teachers to abandon the "lockstep methods of teaching" and substitute individualized instruction. Although he acknowledged that "much has been written and much can yet be said" about individualized instruction, Groszmann was not optimistic about its rapid implementation in the American school system. He based this dour opinion on a conviction that "the difficulties in the way of improving the system are . . . largely financial ones" (p. 90).

Newman (1908), who was more pragmatic than Groszmann, searched for an economical method of spreading individualized instruction in the schools. Newman was a special education teacher who had become somewhat of a celebrity. Although she was flattered by this reputation, she conceded that it was not based on her use of ingenious strategies. In fact, Newman admitted that she "had no particular method of teaching my slow pupils except that I made things very simple and did not give the pupil work that was too difficult for him to understand" (p. 515). Newman recognized that most of the special education teachers who were championing individualized instruction had abandoned drilling, board work, and other labor-saving classroom practices. Disagreeing with their decision, Newman gave examples of ways in which drilling and board work could be reconciled with individualized instruction. She wrote confidently that "I gave a good deal of drill work at the board, which children always enjoy, and which is very helpful in enabling the whole class to progress well" (p. 516). One of Newman's favorite strategies was to encourage her children to work cooperatively during the drills and the board exercises.

Arthur Holmes (1912), who was a Rhode Island superintendent, wrote a text that he christened with an unwieldy subtitle: *A Book for School Executives and Teachers, Being an Exposition of Plans that Have Been Evolved to Adapt School Organization to the Needs of Individual Children, Normal, Supernormal and Subnormal.* Within this book, Holmes described a model of instruction that had been developed by the teachers in Batavia, New York.

> There was an over-crowded [*sic*] room of some sixty pupils in one of the Batavia schools. . . . It was decided to relieve the congestion by putting an additional teacher into the room instead of taking a class out. This teacher . . . was not an assistant to the room teacher. Her rank was co-ordinate but her work was entirely different. It was to be wholly with those pupils who for one reason or another were behind their class. She was to work with these pupils individually until they were able to work with the other members of the class. She was to work with the laggards until they were able to work with the leaders. (p. 74)

Holmes demonstrated flexibility and commitment to individualized instruction throughout his book. For example, he counseled teachers that "almost any of the new 'combination methods' of teaching reading can be used in the auxiliary schools with success" (p. 81).

Arthur Holmes (1912) had exhibited a pragmatic attitude toward reading instruction. He exhibited a comparably pragmatic attitude toward mathematics instruction. His pragmatism was evident when he disagreed with those teachers who categorically discouraged the use of manipulated aids during mathematics exercises. Furthermore, Holmes did not think that these manipulated learning aids had to be abandoned once the students had reached a certain age. Holmes suggested that "the large frame, splints, blocks, squares and other teaching appliances are to be made use of, and their use continued as long as the child needs them" (p. 82).

A year before he had made the preceding remarks, Arthur Holmes (1911) had written about the expanding role of psychology in the schools. The universities that trained teachers were responsible for this expansion. Holmes recounted that "most of the larger institutions of learning in this country . . . [had] taken part in developing a new type of psychology with new content, new methods and new purposes" (p. 11). Pyle (1913), who was a professor at the University of Missouri, also believed that psychology had assumed a greater role in the schools. Pyle wrote that "the gradation of and classification of pupils, methods of teaching and, to a considerable extent, the nature of the curriculum should be based on an accurate knowledge of the mental capacity of the pupils" (p. 61). Pyle judged that the preceding statement was a truism that had been "recognized by everyone who has recently considered the matter" (p. 61). Because he thought so much progress had been made, Pyle stated peremptorily that "we need not take any space" discussing the matter further.

Holmes (1911) and Pyle (1913) had written about the scholastic changes that were transpiring in the first decade of the twentieth century. During that period, Maennel (1909) had published a book about special education. Although Maennel was a German scholar, his work had been translated into English and then marketed by an American publisher. In this influential book, Maennel agreed those scholars who thought that the use of psychology in the schools was gaining momentum. However, Maennel stood out from most scholars because of his ability to rephrase educational discourse in ways that were accessible and attractive to parents. Parents must have applauded Maennel when he chastised those educators who had placed "great stress on subject-matter" but given "little attention to the child, whom we have regarded as a sort of little man, instead of as a child with peculiar feelings, emotions, and thoughts of his own" (p. 201). Maennel reassured his readers that some of the distressing scholastic situations that he had described were about to change. Maennel explained that he was so confident because "more than ever before in the history of man, we are taking into consideration the individual capacities and abilities of our pupils" (p. 201).

Many educators and scholars encouraged teachers to study the backgrounds of individual students and then use these data to customize instruction. Tredgold (1908), a British physician, underscored the value of this procedure. He advised educators that "no success will be attained unless the child's interest is aroused, and this must be the teacher's first care" (p. 337). Dawson (1909) stipulated that "the approach to the problem of the backward child is fundamentally a psychological approach" (p. 430). As such, Dawson recommended that teachers investigate "the ways in which the child primarily acquires its [*sic*] experiences" (p. 430). This classroom information was to be supplemented with data about each student's emotions, health, physical growth, and racial heritage. Dawson wished to call teachers' attention to an overwhelming amount of information. The scope of this information was revealed when he counseled them about a way to analyze a child's "home environment." He wrote that their analysis should include "the number of rooms in the house, whether an upper or lower tenement, or detached house; his street environment; play-life; required occupations; and spontaneous occupations . . . health of parents and other children in the family, food eaten at each meal, and habits of sleep" (p. 431).

Maennel (1909) was another scholar who thought that background inventories could help special educators individualize their instruction. One of the inventories that he reviewed was intended to help the teachers assemble historical profiles of familial illnesses and ancestral disabilities. It also helped them collect information about children's nutritional habits, physical development, intellectual development, and ethical irregularities. With regard to ethical irregularities, this questionnaire helped teachers ascertain whether children exhibited "evidence of any special defects or abnormal tendencies as, for example, lying, fear, appetite (gluttony), [and] laziness" (passage from a background questionnaire developed by M. Görke, n.d., as quoted by Maennel, 1909, p. 95).

The questionnaire to which Maennel (1909) had referred was to be administered by teachers. However, it was to be accompanied by a separate inventory that physicians would complete. The second inventory was a record of children's physical, emotional, and intellectual health. Each section of the report was extremely specific. For example, the section on children's intellectual health directed physicians to gather information about speed of thought, grammar, attention, imagination, memory, judgment, reasoning, and the ways in which the child conceptualized number, form, color, time, and space. Once the teacher's inventory and the physician's inventory were completed, the teacher was to compile a special document that summarized the information from both of them. This document was "to be carried along by the teacher during the whole of the child's school career" (background questionnaire developed by M. Görke, n.d., as quoted by Maennel, 1909, p. 97). Although it already should have been evident to teachers, Maennel advised them that this comprehensive approach to recordkeeping entailed "much work in writing" (p. 93).

Maennel (1909) was one of the many European educators who influenced American scholars and teachers. Lapage (1911), who was another influential scholar, had written about special education in the public schools of Great Britain. As far as the classrooms in which instruction would transpire, Lapage thought that these rooms should not "be too bright and pretty" (p. 271). Despite these restrictions, Lapage believed that "plenty of light, plenty of warmth, and plenty of floor-space" were necessary.

Lapage (1911) also gave advice about learning activities. He recommended that some of these activities be conducted in a special "sense-room."

> [The sense-room contains] large tables which stand out from the wall into the centre [*sic*] of the room. There is one for each of the five senses; [*sic*] sight, smell, hearing, taste and touch. Against the walls are labeled cupboards for the necessary articles with which to test and train the child's senses. Thus, there are in the sight-cupboard a variety of objects, similar to the usual kindergarten bricks and models, but made at least three times larger than these. The brick is six inches in length by one inch square; the cones are six inches high; all are made on this scale. There is a great variety of models and all are gaudily coloured [*sic*] in the primary colours [*sic*] and are made in duplicate. . . . The child stands at the table, on which the different

> models are set out; he is given, say, a red brick; it is large enough for him to grasp it easily and bright enough for him to see it clearly. He is told to move around the table until he finds another model exactly in shape and colour [*sic*]. If he be given a red star he must find another red star and bring it to the teacher and fit it into the star-shaped hole in the piece of wood from which it was cut. (p. 272)

The materials and activities that were described in the preceding passage were intended to appeal to a learner's visual sense. Lapage described equally creative materials and activities for stimulating the other four senses.

Even though the sense-room may have seemed eccentric to his contemporaries, Lapage (1911) championed its use. He recommended many other atypical but extremely pragmatic materials. For example, he encouraged classroom teachers to use "strands of red and yellow and blue cloth, hanging from hooks on the wall, ready for plaiting" (p. 274). He though these devices were worthwhile because the students "have to reach up a very little to get at them, and the attitude is a good one for the feeble-minded, whose inclination is too often to look down and hang the head" (p. 274).

Many American educators were inspired by the individualized special education programs that the Europeans had devised. The Europeans even provided practical advice about ways of initiating an individualized instructional program. For example, De Sanctis (1911) recommended that educators begin the process by using both medical and pedagogical criteria to differentiate children with disabilities. With regard to pedagogy, De Sanctis thought that children with severe disabilities should go to asylums or special hospitals, where the staffs would prescribe the peculiar form of individualized training that those children needed. However, he recommended that children with mild or moderate disabilities attend special schools. Aware that some parents of children with mild or moderate disabilities would not have access to a special school, De Sanctis adjured them to search for an asylum-based program that was accepting "day pupils."

Green (1911; 1912), who was British, was a cotemporary of De Sanctis. Like De Sanctis, he was a proponent of individualized instruction. Green expressed special admiration for those pioneering scholars who "had adopted special methods" to help students with disabilities. To place the German initiatives in perspective, Green contrasted special education in Germany with that in Great Britain. He judged that the administrators and teachers in the German schools had done a superior job of focusing attention and resources on learners' individual needs. As for the British school administrators, Green concluded that they had been "content to let the problem of the backward child remain with the struggling teacher, who can, in general do nothing more for him than insist upon his repeating the meaningless grind at which he has previously failed" (1911, p. 158).

Like many American educators, Morgan (1914) admired her European peers. Morgan wrote a book about special education that she subtitled *A Practical Manual for Teachers and Students*. The appropriateness of this subtitle seemed to be validated after she developed an entire chapter on pedagogy. This chapter, which was peppered with medical, legal, and educational jargon, emphasized the need to individualize instruction. This emphasis should have been apparent to readers after they had perused the opening paragraph.

> It is evident that when one goes about making a diagnosis, one cannot hold a brief [*sic*] for any single kind of training as a cure-all. One must be as impartial in choosing the remedy as in looking for the disease. The individual difficulty is the thing, and any device, fantastic or obvious, which tends to remove that difficulty, is the only cure worth considering. (p. 197)

Morgan's approach to instruction had been highly individualized but also extremely directive. It was quite distinct from the individualized approaches that progressive educators had championed during this era. The progressive educators, such as Italy's Maria Montessori and America's John Dewey, had attempted to nurture children's native abilities. They resisted the temptation to impose structure on students' learning. In a series of articles that she wrote for *McClure's Magazine*, Tozier (1911a; 1911b; 1912) highlighted the "absence of imposed structure" as the key feature of progressive programs. Tozier actually characterized Maria Montessori's instructional method as an instance of "auto-education." At the beginning of the twentieth century, a philosophical chasm separated the proponents of progressive education from the proponents of special education. Throughout the twentieth century, this chasm continued to divide the two groups.

Anticipating that special educators might be overwhelmed by the expectation that they individualize all of their instruction, Morgan reassured them that this procedure would not be onerous. She wrote that "backward children can be brought up to a moral average in their lessons by half an hour's daily individual training" (1914, p. 197). Furthermore, Morgan believed that a limited type of individualized instruction could be delivered by staff members who were not special educators. She suggested that these staff members "may even be inexperienced, provided only the diagnosis has been made by a competent examiner and the directions given by her for training are clear-cut and specific" (pp. 197–198). To promote this type of collaboration, Morgan advised special educators to avoid "elaborate material" or "unusual methods" and rely instead on "the things that a child does every day" (p. 198). Morgan then gave numerous examples of lessons that adhered to her guidelines.

Not all special educators agreed with Morgan (1914) about the value of inexperienced classroom personnel. Witmer (1915), who was a professor of education at the University of Pennsylvania, thought only specialists could deliver individualized education.

> I believe there is a career within the filed of education open to psychologically trained teachers, whose professional training should be superimposed upon a four year [*sic*] college course or its equivalent. This expert teacher is to be a trainer of backward children, i.e. restoration cases, and other classes of children whose education treatment may be put on an individual basis. (p. 226)

Arthur Holmes (1915) was another educator who attempted to solve some of the practical problems that the demand for individualized instruction had created. He reassured teachers who were planning to individualize instruction that they could minimize their efforts. For example, they could consolidate the scheduling of scholastic activities. The use of a common schedule would enable them to prepare lessons collaboratively. It also would enable them to supervise students collaboratively. Holmes illustrated a common schedule with which special educators could organize the first half of each school day.

> 9:00–9:15—Opening exercises all together.
>
> 9:15–9:30—Morning talk to all.
>
> 9:30–9:45—Written language.
>
> 9:45–10:00—Paper language.
>
> 10:00–10:15—Number.
>
> 10:15–10:30—Relaxation.
>
> 10:30–11:00—Manual work.
> 11:00–11:30—Number.
>
> 11:30–12:30—Gymnasium and pool. (p. 237)

More and more educators began to acclaim the value of individualized instruction. Witmer (1916), who was a professor of psychology at the University of Pennsylvania, exemplified this tendency. After presenting a detailed case study, Witmer concluded that the failure of teachers to individualize pedagogy for the student in question had contributed to "a record of very considerable backwardness" (p. 185). He wrote firmly that "I do think that in the educational backwardness of this boy, one factor is a faulty educational method" (p. 191). To correct the situation, Witmer recommended an educational program that would be tailored to the student's aptitudes rather than his weaknesses.

Sunne (1917), who was a professor at Newcomb College in New Orleans, was convinced of the value of individualized instruction. Unlike most of his contemporaries, Sunne focused his attention on the performance of children who were disabled and who represented diverse social groups. After analyzing this performance, he detected racial implications. For example, Sunne reported that the African American children had demonstrated distinctive learning skills. Therefore, he suggested that teachers of African American children refrain from "exclusively trying to fit them into the pattern that suits a majority of the white children" (p. 83). As an alternative, teachers could "encourage and train these peculiar tendencies as well as more general capacities" (p. 83). The manner in which Sunne qualified his own advice revealed his rigorous scientific training. He cautiously advised readers that "the educational bearing" of his advice might turn out to "be significant if corroborated by more extensive investigations" (p. 83).

American Pedagogy During the 1920s

Writing at the very beginning of the twentieth century, Lawrence (1900) had been an articulate advocate for individualized instruction. He had written that "the line between feeble-mindedness and normal-mindedness is not a fixed affair; [*sic*] that feebleminded is a relative state or condition; [*sic*] that there is as much difference between two feeble-minded children as there is between two children in the grades" (p. 100). Lawrence concluded that children with disabilities and those without them would benefit from individualized instruction. During the first two decades of the twentieth century, more and more special educators began to agree with Lawrence. This trend, which continued throughout the 1920s, was reflected in testimonials from professionals.

In 1921, a professor at Yale University investigated the special educational services that were available in New Haven, Connecticut. Disappointed with the current situation, the professor (Gesell, 1921) gave the local school administrators suggestions. He advised them to establish a program that encompassed accurate diagnoses, appropriate instructional placements, vocational guidance, and a system of lifelong support. He emphasized that the program he had in mind would incorporate an individualized educational approach. Although this professor advised the New Haven administrators that they eventually should train their own personnel, he adjured them to start by hiring teachers who were qualified to "initiate and supervise individual programs for educationally exceptional children in regular classrooms" (p. 54).

Within a book about pedagogy, Hollingworth (1923) also emphasized the need for special educators to individualize instruction. She made this point while discussing "word-blind" students. Hollingworth explained that these were students who had "nothing wrong with the visual apparatus" but who still demonstrated "inferiority in reading" (p. 63). Hollingworth thought that the research on word blindness was especially important because it "calls attention to the needs of such children, and shows that they can be taught" (p. 65). She added that those word-blind students who had learned to read were successful because their teachers had recognized "the necessity of individual teaching" (p. 65).

Hollingworth's book had been part of a series of educational monographs produced by the Macmillan publishers. In the introduction to this book, the series editor (O'Shea, 1923) characterized Hollingworth as a scholar who was aware of the "differences among individuals in ability" and who used this knowledge to present "in detail what is known to-day [*sic*] regarding special talents and defects as revealed in the more important subjects taught in the schools" (p. xviii). In the same year that Macmillan's editor had made the preceding remarks, Woodrow (1923) published an extremely practical book for special educators. The practicality of the book was demonstrated in the 35-page chapter on pedagogy. In the opening sentence of that chapter, Woodrow explained that effective teachers "adapt education to individual differences" and then apply "the proper education methods for use with different classes and different individuals within these classes" (p. 275).

Individually instructing students with disabilities had advantages that were relatively easy to appreciate. However, it had a major disadvantage: it raised the cost of special education. That cost increased even further when individualized instruction was combined with other educational innovations. For example some educators, such as Wallin (1933), had suggested that individualized education should be combined with vocational training and then offered to elementary-school students. Before they could implement these sorts of recommendations, school administrators had to provide teachers with special training. They also had to provide them with specific types of equipment and supplies. Figure 3.5 represents some of materials that Wallin thought teachers would need in order to commence instruction about shoe repair (p. 152).

Because special education encumbered significant supplies, equipment, facilities, and personnel, some critics complained that it was undermining the education of talented students. To substantiate this charge, they adduced evidence of declining academic achievement in the schools. Inskeep (1926), who described herself as a "specialist in the teaching of atypical children," acknowledged the difficulty of refuting this charge. However, she still insisted that special education was not responsible for the

Shoe Repair Supplies & Equipment

Awls, pegging, regular, haft, pat. Reg.	Each
Dye, Eddy's in 4 oz. bottles —brown, —black	Bottle
Edge shave, hand adjust-able	Each
Hammer, Rex No. 2	Each
Knives, straight. Curved lip, right hand, 4". Curved lip, left hand, 4"	Each
Lasting Nippers	Each
Leather, cut stock for sol-ing, No. 1, 4¾, 1 doz to pkg. Scrap for practice soling, large pieces	Doz.
Nail set, 1/16"	Each
Nails, in 1 lb. pkgs. 4/8 Channel, 19; ⅝, 6/8, ⅞, Heel, 15, 6/8, 13	Lb.
Pinches, large	Each
Rasp, Crispin, 8"	Each
Stand, with 4 lasts, 24"	Each
Tacks, shoe, in lb. Pkgs. No. 1, 2, 3	Pkg.

Figure 3.5. Early Twentieth-Century List of Some of the Vocational Equipment and Supplies Required by Special Educators.

decline in academic achievement. In the foreword to her textbook about special education, Inskeep suggested two other reasons why "it has been difficult to maintain the average standard of attainment which formerly held for the rank and file of children attending school" (p. x). Inskeep explained "that we have increased our demands for compulsory education . . . so that there is a persistence of the inept minds all through the grades" (p. x). Additionally, she believed that "a great many of our foreigners are not of average mental stock" (p. x). Returning several years later to her second point, Inskeep (1930) reasoned that "the most intelligent stratum of society in any country does not, as a rule, migrate in large numbers" (p. 305). Inskeep was especially worried about the children of immigrants from "Southern Europe, the Azores, Mexico, and other lands where education has not been compulsory" (1930, p. 305).

Although she did not agree with Inskeep's explanation for declining academic achievement, Descoeudres (1928) did agree with her that critics had been blaming special education. Descoeudres wrote that the public had begun to question the funneling of "so much money and effort—including in many cases the flower of the teaching profession—to children who will never pull more than half their weight in society" (p. 13). After paraphrasing the remarks from hostile critics, Descoeudres made an ingenious repartee. She argued that special education could benefit the entire educational system. She explained that "the study of the mental abnormalities of defectives, and the almost insuperable difficulties that ordinary teaching presents to them, will enable us to put our finger on the weaknesses and defects of modern teaching" (p. 14). For this reason, "more than one competent educator" had recommended that "all who intend to become teachers should spend a certain amount of time with the mentally defective" (p. 15).

Cornell and Ross (1928) agreed with Descoeudres that special education should become "an integral part of the educational system" (p. 83). They urged school administrators to accept the responsibility "to care for children whose ability is inadequate to the demands of the regular curriculum" (p. 83). Cornell and Ross thought that this care would require a curriculum with a practical orientation. To clarify this point, they gave examples of the types of skills that special education students should develop in arithmetic, reading, and social studies. In the case of arithmetic, the students were to "know how to deposit money in a bank and how to draw checks; they should realize the advantage of interest bearing accounts; they should have sufficient drill in the fundamental operations to give them skill in solving the life problems which will confront them" (p. 87). In reading, students were to "learn where to find news items of interest, 'help wanted' advertisements, the 'lost and found' column, the sports page, [and] food and clothing advertisements" (p. 87). In social studies, the students were to learn about "the out-patient department of the local hospital, the health department, the child-welfare bureau, the legal aid bureau, [and] the police department" (p. 88). After characterizing the preceding activities as "academic work of a practical sort," Cornell and Ross judged that they were "becoming more and more wide spread" (p. 87).

Summary

Although most of their colleagues believed that students with disabilities were an amorphous group, some American scholars disagreed. They thought that these students should be sorted into precise categories and then instructed on the basis of their distinctive abilities and disabilities. Their approach certainly was economical. It also seemed to be effective. However, it was so sophisticated that even some of its most ardent proponents did not have the skill to put it into practice. Searching for simple-to-implement alternatives, they adapted techniques that European educators already had refined. These techniques enabled them to assess students, manage classrooms, develop curricula, and individualize instruction.

4

Vocational Education

The employment of insane persons should, as far as it is practicable, be adapted to their previous habits, inclinations, and capacities, and . . . the greatest benefit will . . . be found to result from the patient being engaged in that employment in which he can most easily excel.

—Tuke, 1815b

Some members of the public wished to send disabled adults to group homes. They pointed out that these facilities were comfortable, inexpensive, and able to accommodate many of the patients that the asylums had turned away. The staffs at the group homes encouraged the residents to help with chores or assume jobs. They believed that employment presented opportunities to implement therapy and reduce operating costs. However, they recognized that few of their patients were prepared for employment. Therefore, they turned to vocational education. They simultaneously encouraged educators to introduce special vocational training into the public schools.

Early European Vocational Training

Even though the early reformers were confident that special education was worthwhile, they looked for an opportunity to increase its effectiveness. They hoped that vocational training might be that opportunity. Samuel Tuke (1815b), who had implemented vocational training in British asylums, assured reformers that this innovative treatment had value. He advised a group of Americans who were designing an asylum to follow his example and make vocational training a "leading feature of the new institution" (p. 7).

To emphasize the value of vocational training, Samuel Tuke (1815b) recounted details about the patients at a Spanish asylum. He noted that these patients had represented several social strata. Those patients from the lower social ranks had assumed jobs. In contrast, those patients who were members of the Spanish nobility had been exempted from employment. After he had analyzed the rehabilitation of the patients, Tuke reported that most of those who eventually were released had been employed. Aware of the similarities between the social structures of Spain and Great Britain, Tuke exercised caution when he was delineating the implications of this research. He observed diplomatically that the obvious benefits of employment-based therapy did not justify its use with every patient. He explained that "where the reluctance on the part of the patient is great, the irritation which compulsory means are likely to excite, will probably be more injurious to the patient, than the exercise will be beneficial" (p. 7).

Samuel Tuke (1815b) had discerned ways in which adults with disabilities could benefit from vocational activities. However, he noted that these activities had advantages for the staff members at asylums as well as for the patients. Tuke wrote that "many of the women may, with equal economy to the Institution and benefit to themselves, be employed in assisting the servants and nurses" (p. 44). Tuke also was sure that the male patients could provide some institutional payback. He wrote that they could perform "a great part of the out-of-doors work" (p. 44). Tuke quickly added that all work by patients was to be conducted "under the care of a judicious director."

Daniel Tuke, who was the son of Samuel Tuke, shared his father's passion to help disabled persons. He also shared his father's convictions about the value of vocational education. Daniel Tuke (1875) wrote about a British asylum at which vocational education had been used extensively. He tallied the multiple types of vocational training activities to which the 1039 patients at this asylum had been assigned.

> *Men*—Garden and farm labourers [*sic*], 90; assisting servants to clean house, 65; miscellaneous employment, 27; shoemaking, 12; tailoring, 11; painting, 5; carpentry, 8. *Women*—Needlework 114; assisting servants, 67; miscellaneous, 33; assisting in laundry, 55; knitting, 15; quilting, 9; fancy work 1. (Italics as in the original, p. 2)

Both Samuel Tuke and Daniel Tuke had detected opportunities for persons with disabilities to work. The superintendents of several asylums agreed with them. More and more employers also agreed with them. Toward the middle of the nineteenth century, Arlidge (1859) noted that persons with disabilities were being assigned routinely to "workhouse detention" programs as well as asylums. Attempting to convey the scope of this practice, Arlidge estimated that half of the persons currently housed in workhouses would qualify for admission to asylums. Believing that these detainees would have had better lives in asylums, Arlidge protested that the "insane in the workhouses should rightly enjoy the advantages of the supervision, general management, nursing, and dietary of asylums" (p. 26). He thought that recent publicity about the exploitation of the disabled persons in workhouses had created some opposition to this practice. However, Arlidge pointed out that the roots of this problem were politically entangled. For example, some community leaders had been sending individuals to workhouses even though they knew that those individuals were unable to engage in labor. These community leaders had recognized that these assignments had not been in the best interests of persons with disabilities. Arlidge explained that they had persevered with the placements primarily because of "the much greater cheapness of workhouse compared with asylum detention" (p. 40).

Down (1876), who was a British physician, was convinced that vocational education was valuable to persons with disabilities. In fact, he wrote that the "primary object" of special education was "to make the pupil self-helpful and, as far as possible, a useful working member of the community" (p. 16). To ensure that his readers did not miss this important point, he added that "mere abstract . . . knowledge is of little value," and that "everything which makes [the student] useful makes him proportionately happy" (p. 16). Down gave a detailed example of the ways in which vocational skills could be nurtured.

> The uses and value of money, and the value and weight of commodities is [*sic*] best taught by a plan which I have devised of instituting a shop, furnished with the usual appliances of sale. One patient acts as the customer and another as the trader. In this way a purchase is effected [*sic*], and the whole transaction of weighing, calculating, and paying is made under the criticism of an assembled class. (p. 15)

Worried that the preceding scenario could be too cerebral for some learners, Down suggested that teachers occasionally substitute gardening activities for the shopping activities. He explained that this variable pattern was desirable so that "the physical may alternate with the intellectual training" (p. 16).

Ireland (1877) was another nineteenth-century British physician who made pioneering efforts on behalf of persons with disabilities. Like Down, he was a strong advocate of vocational education. Although he did not conceal his enthusiasm for this approach, Ireland faithfully pointed out its controversial features. For example, he noted that some individuals had questioned the usefulness of vocational education because they thought that disabled persons were "naturally indolent." An additional drawback was the inordinate amount of time that the training of persons with disabilities required. With reference to this last point, Ireland conceded that five or six years were "usually required for an ordinary apprenticeship" (p. 354). Although he did not dismiss these criticisms, Ireland provided a philosophical rejoinder. Shifting the dialogue to a humanitarian plane, he observed that "once [persons with disabilities] have fairly learnt [to work], it may fill up many dreary hours in their lives, and may lead to their making their bread, or being very helpful to others" (p. 324).

Members of the public had questioned the types of employment for which disabled persons could be prepared. Ireland (1877) had specific advice on this matter. He recommended that "grown-up imbecile girls" be prepared to look after young children with disabilities. He noted that these women were "much more willing to remain beside the children [than were paid nurses], and many difficulties have been tided over, and many accidents have been avoided, by their affectionate care" (p. 355). Although Ireland observed that the male patients at some asylums had been taught to manufacture sash cords or cigars, he identified the typical trades in British asylums as "mat-making, brush-making, shoe-making, tailoring, and the cultivation of the ground" (p. 324).

In addition to answering the questions that the critics of vocational education had posed, Ireland (1877) raised his own questions. For example, he asked about the ideal ratio of general training to highly specialized training within a vocational education program. To place this question in perspective, Ireland made several observations about those institutions that were supported by private charity. He judged that the staffs at these institutions had propounded an extremely specialized type of training. Ireland concluded that they had a tendency to "single out a special faculty which is more prominent than the rest, and to try to educate it; forgetting all the others" (p. 323). Ireland worried that the directors of charitable institutions had endorsed this model of training so that they could gather publicity and win the favor of benefactors. For this reason, these directors usually highlighted the accomplishments of select patients. Ireland gave several examples, such as "an idiot who can paint portraits, an idiot who can make models of ships, which look very well out of the water, [and] an idiot who can spell backwards with great rapidity" (p. 323). Ireland speculated that such accomplishments, although they might help to raise funds for charitable institutions, were not in the best interest of the patients. To ensure that his position on this matter was clear, Ireland asked his readers to consider whether a disabled person who was "portrait painter" or a "maker of models" could ever earn a living with those skills. As to the employment prospects for persons who could spell backwards, Ireland did not think that it was necessary to comment on this matter.

Sherlock (1911) was still another British physician who became an advocate for persons with disabilities during the early years of the twentieth century. As the superintendent of a British Asylum, he had initiated several progressive practices. For example, Sherlock had trained disabled persons to discharge household tasks. He then "boarded out" some of these patients to households in the community. One clear advantage of this program was its "cheapness." However, Sherlock believed that the program's economic value had not been fully recognized. He explained that most administrators and employers had underestimated the "earning capacity" of those persons who had been placed in community households.

Although Sherlock (1911) was an advocate of "boarding out," he did recognize that this practice had problems. He speculated about some of these problems.

> It is not easy . . . to find the necessary combination of a good house and a good householder. A working man of the better class, for example, does not want an idiot always about the house, especially if he has children of his own, and anything like adequate inspection is likely to be resented. The risks that the feeble-minded person may injure himself or another, or may give way to drunkenness or sexual malpractices vary inversely as [*sic*] the supervision exercised over him. (p. 271)

Sherlock (1911) believed that the British legislature could solve some of the problems in programs for disabled adults. He urged legislators to restrict the practice of "boarding out" to those group homes at which the patients would receive appropriate care and supervision. To ensure compliance, he recommended that every group home employ a craftsmaster, who "would be responsible for the control of all the male colonists who could be usefully employed" (p. 280). Sherlock explained that the craftsmaster "would have charge of them while they were at leisure and would endeavor, generally, so to order their lives as to make them happy and useful members of the community" (p. 280). Sherlock also recommended that every group home engage a craftsmistress to supervise the female patients.

Early American Vocational Training

Europeans had been the early advocates for special vocational training. However, some Americans did follow their lead. Stewart (1882), who was an educator at a Kentucky school for students with disabilities, reported about the innovative programs at his institution. He wrote that "it has been demonstrated in our institution that *some* children who could not be *taught to read or write could* be taught some useful type of labor" (italics as in the original, p. 237). Stewart pointed out that even those boys of the "lowest grade have shown an aptness for tying brooms or making mops or stuffing and sewing a mattress" (p. 237). In fact, he estimated that 80 percent of the students who had been admitted to this school had the aptitude to be self-supporting. Stewart gave examples of persons who had learned trades and then been "adopted into homes, where they are well cared for and receive wages" (pp. 236–237). He also gave examples of institutional graduates who had assumed salaried jobs and become financially independent.

Despite his enthusiasm for the way in which vocational education was taught in the Kentucky program, Stewart (1882) did provide two cautions about the graduates of that program. He noted that none of them had been appointed as supervisors at their work sites. Furthermore, he believed that none of them would "ever be foremen in their specialty" (p. 239). After he had made these concessions, Stewart (1882) still insisted that "under the guidance of competent men, their skill will always command such wages as will enable them to live without aid or help from any source, and keep them out of path usually sought by the idle and vicious" (p. 239).

Writing during the same decade as Stewart, Barrows (1888) reported on a resolution that had been adopted by the Association of American Institutions for the Idiotic and Feeble-minded. He quoted the actual language of that resolution.

> [The members resolve that:] For those of school-attending age, institutions should be provided with properly equipped school departments, especially with a view of developing the enfeebled mental faculties, and training them to habits of industry. That by these means a very large proportion can be made useful and helpful to themselves or others. Many will become partially self-supporting, and a lesser number entirely so. . . . That for the adult portion, with a mental capacity sufficient for the performance of labor, farms and shops should be added, and industries established and maintained, that their labor may be utilized for the benefit of the State. (Resolution adopted by the Association of American Institutions for the Idiotic and Feeble-minded, 1888, as reported by Barrows, 1888, p. 395)

Barrow (1888) personally endorsed the preceding resolution. He tried to win the support of his readers with an anecdote.

> A short time ago a painter went out, who was not what Dr. Byers would call "a six-button kid-glove idiot." He was rather of the lower order, yet with a wonderful power of application and industry. The thing that he had learned was painting. He went out and got two dollars and a quarter a day. His employer paid him more than he was paying his other strong-minded, whole-minded men, [*sic*] because he was so steady and had no bad habits. (p. 399)

Rogers (1888) was a Minnesota physician and the editor-in-chief of the *Journal of Psycho Asthenics*. He described some of the nineteenth-century programs that had been designed to help disabled persons master vocational skills. He reported that these programs had been so successful that "scores of feeble-minded persons are to-day performing the work of regular employees in public institutions, and might under favorable circumstances earn a livelihood outside" (p. 102). However, Rogers did admit the difficulty he had encountered while attempting to find "outside" employment for workers with disabilities. He advised colleagues who intended to replicate his program that they should anticipate comparable difficulties.

> This is a busy, practical, money-getting age, when the satisfactory placing of children of normal faculties is no easy task, and only under favorable circumstances to be advised. This being true of normal persons, how small the field for those lacking in judgment and the higher qualifications for success! (p. 102)

Despite his warning about the difficulty of securing extra-asylum jobs, Rogers identified vocational education as one of the "most important" services that institutional administrators could offer patients. He wrote that the administrators should go as "far as possible" in their efforts to transform patients into "self-supporting members of society" (1888, p. 101).

Salisbury (1892) presented details about the special vocational programs that he had visited. These programs had been established at residential schools in Illinois and Minnesota. In a report that he made to the Wisconsin State Teachers' Association, Salisbury noted that the students' schoolwork was "preceded, relieved, and supplemented by industrial training, sewing, and needle-work for the girls, mechanical and agricultural activity for the boys" (p. 226). Salisbury elaborated on the vocational activities of the male students.

> In both the institutions visited the farm and garden have been found most useful and profitable adjuncts, furnishing suitable and healthful occupation to many of the inmates, even those of too low a type to receive much benefit from the school agencies. In the Minnesota institution, brush-making has been developed into a helpful in-door [*sic*] industry. In the Illinois institution, shoemaking is carried on to some extent, as also tailoring; wood-carving and repoussé-work [*sic*] in brass furnish more artistic outlets of activity. (p. 226)

With regard to the pedagogy that should guide the education of youths with disabilities, Salisbury (1892) observed that "the same principles of education are valid here as elsewhere" (p. 226). For example, he suggested that all learning activities should "be highly individualized." Salisbury added that "there is unlimited room and need for special skill and sagacity in their application to the infinitely varying conditions" (p. 226). He concluded by admonishing teachers to apply these principles with "patience, insight, and ingenuity" (p. 226).

Walter Fernald (1893) described the extent to which vocational education had been embedded into some nineteenth-century American asylums.

> In the institution [for persons with disabilities] the boys assist the baker, carpenter, and engineer. They do much of the shoemaking, the tailoring, and the painting. They drive teams, build roads, and dig ditches. Nearly all of the institutions have large farms and gardens, which supply enormous quantities of milk and vegetables for the consumption of the imamates [*sic*]. . . . The females do the laundry work, make the clothing and bedding, and do a large share of all the other domestic work of these immense households. Many of these adult females, naturally kind and gentle, have the instinctive feminine love for children, and are of great assistance caring for the feeble and crippled children in the custodial department. (p. 218)

After he had illustrated some of the ways in which vocational education had been implemented, Walter Fernald (1893) gave several reasons for its increasing popularity.

> The daily routine work in a large institution furnishes these trained adults with abundant opportunities for doing simple manual labor, which otherwise would have to be done by paid employees. Outside of an institution it would be impossible to secure the experienced and patient supervision and direction necessary to obtain practical, remunerative results from the comparatively unskilled labor of these feeble-minded people. . . . The average running expenses of these institutions have been gradually and largely reduced by this utilization of the industrial abilities of the trained inmates. (pp. 218–219)

Wilbur (1888), who was a physician at a Michigan school for persons with disabilities, agreed with those European scholars who had placed a high value on vocational education. However, he questioned whether vocational education should be represented as the road to independence. Wilbur professed this skepticism even though he believed that "the capacity of the individual [with disabilities] is not at fault" (p. 110). He used an illustration to clarify his point.

> Take the case of the feeble-minded female, who has been educated in an institution to be an expert in many of the domestic employments: how can she be sent out into the world to seek employment, without careful protection and guardianship? I have in mind a female of this class, who is well developed in form and fair of features, an inmate of the Illinois asylum, who was a first-class ironer. I know, too, where her services would bring her the very best of wages,—enough [*sic*] to sustain her independently and well,—but [*sic*] I would never advocate placing her in the situation I refer to. It would be unjustifiable with the surroundings connected with it. (p. 110)

Wilbur carefully chose prose to ensure that his readers understood his sentiments on this matter. He advised them that "the world is not full of philanthropic people who are willing to take the individual from the asylum and surround him with the proper guardianship which his case demands" (p. 110).

Early Twentieth-Century American Efforts

Lawrence (1900) was skeptical about the effectiveness of special vocational training. He was skeptical even though these programs created "good workers" who were "very sensitive to neglect or personal reference" (p. 107). Lawrence even conceded that "many quite feeble-minded children would be self-supporting in the outside world" (p. 107). Although he appreciated disabled workers' talents, Lawrence thought that few of them could gain extra-institutional employment. One reason for this difficulty was that disabled workers frequently exhibited "some unpleasant peculiarity of face or form" (p. 107). Convinced that many disabled workers would be unable to "find a place to sell their services for even food and clothing in the outside world," Lawrence suggested that they be restricted to asylums, where they could "care for those children below their own grade" (p. 107).

Johnstone (1898), who was an administrator at an Indiana institution for students with disabilities, believed that vocational education did promote student independence. However, he conceded this point reluctantly. Johnstone indicated that that he had "no desire to make our [special] child self-directing" (p. 98). Instead of encouraging them toward independence, he wished to convince special learners that they "must always be under the direction of the institution" (p. 98). Johnstone added that "what *we* do wish is, to make him as nearly self-supporting as possible in the institution" (italics as in the original, p. 98). Johnstone was aware that universal, life-long institutionalization had been criticized as too expensive. Wishing to address this criticism, Johnstone pointed to one way in which institutionalization was economical. He explained that any child who could work in an institution, and thereby help reduce the institutional responsibilities of paid employees, was, in effect, "contributing so much towards his own support" (p. 98).

Dunphy (1908), who was the superintendent for the New York City schools on Randall's Island, was concerned about the political movement to promote independence among disabled persons. Even though she was writing more than a decade after Johnstone (1898) had made remarks on this subject, she still agreed with him about the grave dangers of this plan. To make her case, Dunphy posed a question to her readers. She asked them whether the education of children with disabilities could be "in a small measure" comparable to the education of children who were normal. Responding to her own question, she noted that "to a limited degree and under certain well-defined conditions, we may answer yes to the above query" (p. 326). However, Dunphy immediately added a stipulation.

> We can render the defective socially efficient and comparatively self-reliant, provided we confine his efforts at usefulness within the sphere of a community of his mental equals. It would be futile to assert that any amount of training will sufficiently develop the defectives to a point of usefulness that will enable them to cope with the problems of the world at large, and it would be manifestly unjust to exact from him the same measure of mental poise demanded of the normal human being. (pp. 326–327)

Dunphy concluded that the education of persons with disabilities "should rest on a definite, practical basis, as it is only by constant employment . . . that an economic return for the time, care and expense necessary to develop defectives to a point of usefulness can be obtained" (p. 327).

Some American educators did not believe that special vocational training would liberate dangerous persons. Therefore, they disregarded the warnings about it. These educators admired the European training model in which disabled persons were prepared for independent living. Allen (1904) reviewed the nineteenth-century training models for students who were visually impaired. He concluded that "industrial training has been an integral part of the course [of preparation] from the beginning" (p. 791). To highlight the ways in which vocational education had enhanced the effectiveness of these programs, Allen listed some of the popular trades that visually impaired students had mastered. These trades included chair-caning, hammock-making, broom-making, and carpet-weaving. Allen noted that "before the introduction of such varieties of labor-saving machinery as the last half century has seen, many of the discharged pupils followed some manual trade and succeeded in subsisting by it" (p. 791). Allen regretted that "today this is less and less possible" (p. 791).

Chace (1904) had indicated that she admired the special education programs that British educators had established. She noted that the youngsters who had been attending the British schools included "not merely dull or backward" students but also those who were "incapable of receiving proper benefit in the ordinary public elementary schools" (passage from Britain's *Epileptic Act of 1899*, as quoted by Chace, 1904, p. 393). As for goals that American educators should adopt, Chace recommended that they aspire to help each student "become self-supporting when he leaves school" (p. 401). As to methods that would expedite this goal, she concluded summarily that "too great emphasis . . . cannot be placed on manual training" (p. 401).

Like Chace, Rosenfeld (1906) discerned ways in whish vocational education could help American learners become independent. After visiting 15 schools that were offering special education classes in New York City, Rosenfeld described vocational learning activities that had been implemented. Some of these activities had been introduced into the elementary schools as well as the secondary schools.

> An exaggeration of kindergarten methods is used. The materials for the occupations are all very much enlarged. The children begin with manual work of the simplest kind. It took one child seven months to learn to weave an oil-cloth mat with five colored sticks for strips. . . . The paper weaving can be ultimately used in teaching girls to darn stockings; sewing cards can be the precursors of seams. The children use raffia to make boxes, baskets and picture frames; they also learn woodworking and sewing. (p. 97)

Farrell (1908a) was the administrator in charge of New York City's special education programs. She commented on the special vocational programs that were available to New York City's students.

> Woodwork, with the large tools as opposed to the knife work, gives perhaps the greatest opportunity. The objects made have a real interest for the child since he is allowed to take them home. Towel-rollers, knife-boxes, bread-boards, wheelbarrows, stools, clock-brackets and a dozen other things were made this past year. Clay modeling, bent ironwork, paper-cutting, gardening, basketry and chair-caning are a few of the occupations followed. All the work in this line looks to industrial efficiency. . . . It is our intention to introduce those simple forms of industrial work that the children may follow as a means of earning a living. (pp. 94–95)

Farrell called attention to the positive ways in which parents had reacted to vocational curricula. She recounted that "at an exhibition of work held recently a in [*sic*] public school the parents were surprised at the work done. . . . [and] asked when their child would get in that class so as to learn something useful" (p. 94).

Lobbying by Parents of Special Learners

The parents of children with disabilities wanted to ascertain the best types of education that were available in their communities. Therefore they compared the new vocational programs with the traditional special educational programs. They also compared the special vocational training with the general vocational programs that were available to students without disabilities. After they had completed their analysis, they lobbied the school administrators to ensure that their children were enrolled in the optimal scholastic programs.

Some children with disabilities had been assigned summarily to general vocational schools. Although this practice may have had benefits, it had created political problems. Addams (1914), who was a judge in the juvenile courts of Cleveland, alluded to the frequency with which his judiciary colleagues had been remanding disabled children to regular vocational high schools. These judges had ordered the administrators at vocational schools to make room for the special students. Those school administrators then had to confront the disappointed parents of those children who would have qualified for admission through the competitive application process. The parents protested that judicial placements were depriving their own children of training opportunities. Sympathizing with the disgruntled parents, Addams applauded a new Ohio law. This law had been enacted to facilitate "the removal of sub-normal children from the industrial school . . . and make room for the normal children for whom these schools [*sic*] were planned" (p. 54).

The admission process was not the only aspect of the vocational schools about which parents were concerned. In his report *School Efficiency—A Constructive Study Applied to New York City*, Hanus (1913) adjured school administrators to do a better job of individualizing vocational instruction. Hanus stipulated that "public education should strive to render each pupil economically intelligent and efficient" and to "direct each pupil's attention to a vocation to which he may reasonably aspire" (p. 8). He explained that this adjuration extended to all students. Hanus pointed out that the American people, who were "not satisfied with schools for normal children only," recognized an obligation "to do all that can be done for exceptional children as well" (p. 10). Hanus believed that five categories of students would benefit from special vocational classes. The categories included "mentally defective children." Henry Goddard, a renowned expert on special education, was one of the consultants who had helped Hanus write this report.

Witmer (1915) was a professor at the University of Pennsylvania. He supported vocational education. Furthermore, he staunchly backed those parents who were demanding greater access to special vocational education programs. Even though he backed parents on this issue, Witmer was hardly a proponent of parental empowerment. Aware that many parents of disabled children wanted their youngsters to learn academic skills, he dismissed their requests as unreasonably idealistic. Witmer discouraged academically oriented special education programs because so few of the children were "true restoration cases." He concluded that disabled children lacked the aptitude to lead normal lives. The skeptical Witmer counseled school administrators to hire teachers trained in "manual methods." In fact, he recommended that the preparation of all special educators "be devoted largely, perhaps exclusively, to training in the technique of manual work, dancing, [and] occupations" (p. 224). Witmer lamented that "what one sees all too frequently is a teacher whose training has been primarily academic, engaged in the hopeless task of teaching reading, writing, and arithmetic to children who can never use these processes as tools for their further development" (p. 224).

World War I

During World War I, the public became extremely concerned about the connection between school efficiency and national defense (Giordano, 2004). Employers raised this anxiety further by chastising those school administrators who were not using business models to manage their schools. Looking back on this era, Lazerson and Grubb (1974) noted that the World War I school administrators were pressured to make the schools serve the war effort. Although this political pressure significantly influenced many aspects of the schools, Lazerson and Grubb concluded that "no development was more crucial . . . than vocational education" (p. 1). They explained that the advocates of vocational education were so successful because of their skill in linking vocational education to wartime financial accountability.

Critics believed that those wartime schools that lacked vocational training were inefficient. They even disparaged schools with vocational programs if they did not meet the expectations of industrialists and businesspersons. These school critics were extremely influential. However, their political strength increased after the administrators in the vocational schools began to side with them. For example, Eaton (1917), who was the director of an urban vocational program, challenged the vocations schools in New York City to improve their performance. He wrote that "efficiency, which in the case of all industrial operations means preparedness and standardization, ought to be required of a vocational school as strictly as it is now demanded in modern business" (p. 1). Although he counseled school administrators to ensure that students were learning appropriate skills, Eaton believed that they could improve in other areas as well. Consequently, he instructed the administrators "to record and control the work of the [school] shop in order that production may be facilitated" (p. 1). He thought that they could achieve this goal by closely monitoring "the cost of each operation." If his fellow administrators did not follow his advice, Eaton predicted that their programs would devolve into "slapstick" operations with disadvantages that were "too obvious to require demonstration" (p. 1).

Woolley and Hart (1921) looked back on some of the ways in which persons with disabilities had been employed during the recent war. They called attention to one project in which patients had been released from asylums to work in canneries. Although this project had lasted only a week, Woolley and Hart were impressed because "the morons of the stable type proved able to earn about 75 percent as much on a piece rate basis as normal women who were also beginners" (p. 253). To determine the amount of time that workers with disabilities might remain in jobs, Woolley and Hart examined the participants in another project. They concluded that the males in this second project had kept their jobs for a median period of 11 months. The women in the same project had remained employed for a median period of six months.

Wishing to find still more information about persons with disabilities who had been employed, Woolley and Hart (1921) examined 251 students who had attended special education schools and subsequently secured salaried jobs. The two researchers were interested in the types of jobs for which these students had qualified. They discovered that one hundred and fifty-six of them had become shop or factory workers. Twenty-three of them became messengers, wagon boys, or errand boys. Fourteen became drivers or salespersons. Another six learned to sell newspapers.

During World War I, a perilous international situation had stimulated interest in vocational education. However, American businesspersons also were responsible for the increased interest. They impressed many groups with their testimonials about the effectiveness of vocational programs. Professors comprised still another group that contributed to the rising interest. Douglas (1921), who was a professor of business at the University of Chicago, exemplified many of those professors who had endorsed vocational education. In an article that he had written originally in 1918, he characterized it as "perhaps the most important educational movement of the past decade" (p. 11). Douglas identified economic relevance as the trait that had enabled vocational education to flourish in a wartime environment. Few of his contemporaries would have challenged his appraisal.

Taking Advantage of Reformatories

During the nineteenth century, the public routinely had committed persons with disabilities to reformatories and prisons. Howe (1852) indicated that this practice had been prevalent in Massachusetts during the first half of the twentieth century. He noted that even persons who already had been committed to asylums would be removed "from the only place where they were comfortable, the State lunatic asylum, whenever it was necessary to make room for the less unfortunate insane, and it sent them,—not [*sic*] to another Asylum [*sic*], but to the houses of correction" (p. 4). Howe reported that the Massachusetts legislators enacted a state law in 1846 to curb this practice.

In the early part of the twentieth century, many children with disabilities had been confined in reformatories. Butler (1907) had noted that "mental defectives are frequently committed to the reformatories" and that "in the state prisons, also, are to be found those who are feeble-minded along with others who are epileptics and insane" (p. 5). Some persons supported this type of incarceration because they were convinced that disabled children could not be cured. Some believed that disabled children could not even be helped. Persons with these harsh views saw reformatories as the ideal sites at which to confine youths with disabilities. Milburn (1908) did not conceal his opinion on this matter. He stated that "generally speaking, feeble-mindedness can not be cured" and that "imamates of institutions, practically without exception, are benefited by their residence" (p. 54).

Although Milburn (1908) was adamant about the need to preserve institutionalization, he recognized that many citizens were disconcerted by its high costs. He attempted to change their minds.

> Does [institutionalization in an asylum, prison, or reformatory] pay? The answer to this question is found in that some way or somehow the feeble-minded are sure to be a burden on the public. . . . They may be in jails, they may be in penitentiaries, they may be in almshouses, they may be supported by the overseer of the poor or the charity of neighbors and friends, or in houses of prostitution, spreading contagious disease, but the bill is always sent to the public to pay. (p. 56)

Given his beliefs about the problems that disabled persons created when they were free, Milburn (1908) was sure that reformatories were the appropriate sites at which to detain them. Even many of the individuals who were uncomfortable about reformatories still believed that they could be expedient solutions to complicated social problems. However, the use of reformatories to detain disabled persons created problems of a different sort. For example, Butler (1907) questioned whether many of the persons that were sent to reformatories truly belonged at those sites. He noted that some persons with disabilities had been sent to reformatories only because they had been "nuisances in their respective communities" (p. 5). He judged that others had been detained because of "offenses for which they were not really responsible" (p. 5). Butler thought that still other persons had been committed to reformatories "because there appeared to be no other place to send them" (p. 5). Barr (1902), who was a physician at a Pennsylvania school for children with disabilities, had made similar points. Writing several years before Butler, Barr had observed that only one-tenth of the disabled persons who had been reported in the recent census had been housed in institutions. He noted that the rest had been "scattered through communities" or "filling jails and penitentiaries" (p. 162).

During the second decade of the twentieth century, Johnstone (1916) was concerned that so many disabled persons had been turned away from asylums, hospitals, or special colonies. Instead they had been sent to facilities that he considered inappropriate. As a result, persons with disabilities were being encountered continually by "every worker with the insane and epileptic; the criminal, juvenile delinquents and truants; the syphilitics, prostitutes and other sex offenders; the tramps, paupers and homeless; the drunkards and drug habitues [*sic*]; the inefficients [*sic*] and ne'er-do-wells" (p. 208). In view of the distressing situation, Johnstone counseled educators to extend their efforts to the many disabled persons who were detained in "almshouses and orphanages" or "reformatories and penal institutions" (p. 208).

Barr (1899–1900) had wished to keep disabled patients away from prisons and reformatories. At the same time, he wished to keep them separated from the general populace. Barr was insistent on the latter point. He believed that even those persons with disabilities who appeared to have been successfully "trained" should be sequestered. He warned that "surely history would not write our names among the wise" if society were to "turn these irresponsibles [*sic*] loose to undo the work of the past and redouble that of the future" (p. 211). Although he supported the permanent segregation of all persons with disabilities, Barr recognized the high cost of this plan. He therefore looked to group homes as "the practical solution to this problem." Barr believed that the group homes had financial and humanitarian benefits. As far as their financial value, these homes could be "almost self-supporting" (p. 211). With regard to their humanitarian value, the group homes could have a more positive impact on patients "than the frown of penitentiary walls" (p. 211). Barr wrote that the disabled persons assigned to group homes would be "protected from the world and the world from them" (p. 211). Furthermore, the development of group homes would be a critical milestone in the journey toward "that 'statelier Eden of simple manners, purer laws' which the twentieth century shall usher in" (p. 211).

As one might expect, many of the educators who supported group homes opposed the practice of assigning youths with disabilities to reformatories. However, even some politically conservative educators opposed reformatory placements. In behavior that was just as unpredictable, some progressive educators began to favor reformatory placements. Walter Fernald (1893; 1909), who managed a facility for persons with disabilities in Massachusetts, generally propounded politically progressive policies. Nonetheless, he saw the need to assign some disabled youths to corrective institutions. Walter Fernald explained that "institutions for defectives are often expected to receive patients where the intellectual defect is apparently only moderate, and the principal reasons for institutional treatment is the failure to harmonize with the environment as shown by low tastes and associates" (1909, p. 16). Walter Fernald was sure that some of the patients at his own facility had been classified as disabled solely because of "general incorrigibility, purposeless and needless lying, a quarrelsome disposition, a tendency to petty stealing, a propensity for setting fires, aimless destruction of property, a tendency to run away and lead a life of vagrancy, [and] sexual precocity or perversions" (1909, p. 16).

Van Sickle, Witmer, and Ayres (1911) agreed with Walter Fernald that different types of persons were being classified as disabled. However, they were not upset at this trend. Their distinctive views were apparent in the ways that they defined disabilities. For example, they defined juvenile delinquency through symptoms rather than causes. They specifically associated it with the behaviors of a "group of exceptional children . . . who stood in danger of growing into an adult life of criminality" (p. 9). As far as a cure was concerned, Van Sickle, Witmer, and Ayres endorsed moral training. However, they emphasized that the training should be presented in a nurturing rather than a punitive fashion.

Guy Fernald (1920) was a physician at the Massachusetts Reformatory. Writing after World War I, he indicated that the problem of designating facilities for disabled youths was connected to another problem, namely the inappropriate way in which youths were being classified. He was upset that many disabled youngsters were being sent to reformatories to receive "punitive" treatments. He argued that they actually required "curative" treatments. Guy Fernald thought that this misunderstanding was so widespread that it could not be eliminated without government intervention. He approvingly noted that "public information and sentiment has now reached the point in some of the more progressive states at which legislative action is sought to enable rational treatment" (pp. 161–162). To promote "rational treatment," Guy Fernald recommended special custodial hospitals. These hospitals would serve those youths who were both disabled and delinquent. The hospitalized youths would be separated from their disabled but nondelinquent peers, who would be sent to asylums. The hospitalized youths also would be separated from nondisabled criminals, who would be sent to reformatories.

Vocational Instruction in Reformatories

Many persons thought that vocational training was the most appropriate educational program for youths in reformatories. They judged that it was suitable for incarcerated youths without disabilities as well as those with disabilities. At the beginning of the twentieth century, Snedden (1907) wished to ascertain the prevalence of vocational education in reformatories. He therefore selected an Ohio reformatory to which 823 students had been committed. He then made a detailed study of that institution. Snedden carefully enumerated the many vocational programs to which the students within this school had been assigned. The most popular programs had more than 60 students enrolled in them. These programs included tailoring, farming, and acting as assistants to cottage matrons. Other popular programs were laundering, steam ironing, cooking, table-waiting, clothes-mending, brick-making, printing, and shoe-repairing. Snedden added parenthetically that "none of these industries are remunerative in the sense of bringing in money" but that "very many of them are distinctly profitable in supplying the labor, repairing, and products needed by the institution" (p. 97).

Snedden (1907) had examined the vocational practices at an Ohio institution. The administrators at this institution had not been concerned by the fact that their programs were not generating money. They also had not been concerned that the programs' participants were not earning salaries. Some educators did not share these sentiments. In fact, some reform-school administrators had situated their vocational programs near factories or shops precisely so that their students would take salaried job and generate income. Sometimes this income was kept by the institutions; at other times it was shared with the workers. Maennel (1909) referred to Richter, a German educator who had arranged for students with disabilities to labor as paid interns in mechanical shops. Although he had been somewhat successful, Richter had encountered several problems. One of these problems was the scarcity of employers who were willing to accept disabled workers.

> Would that our master mechanics could be brought to understand that pupils sent out from our auxiliary schools are not nearly as incompetent as people are wont to believe; they are often more capable in practical affairs than boys [*sic*] from the country and elsewhere. (K. Richter, n.d., as quoted by Maennel, 1909, p. 180)

Richter added that the "work of training auxiliary school apprentices pays," but only under those circumstances in which "the master does not leave the matter entirely in the hands of his assistants" (K. Richter, n.d., as quoted by Maennel, 1909, p. 180).

Barr (1902) had implemented vocational programs for persons with disabilities in Pennsylvania. Like Richter, he noted the benefits of these programs. Like Richter, he acknowledged the difficulty of arranging suitable internship sites. Assuming a moralistic vantage, Barr wrote that "the weak-minded is 'hustled' in much the same proportion as his normal brother" (p. 164). He explained that "the vanity of the family or the pressure upon associations" would persuade a disabled male student to quit a vocational training program, even though he had developed only a "smattering of a trade." When a position in a trade school became vacant, one of the many students who were waiting for admission would take that opening. However, Barr was distressed because the newly enrolled student would make the same dysfunctional choices as his predecessor. As a result, the cycle of educational failure would continue.

Hart (1910), who was in charge of "child-helping" for a philanthropic orga-nization, thought that farm-based internships prepared boys for "wholesome and happy" lives. These rural experiences could be especially beneficial to reformatory inmates. However, Hart recognized that the farming internships created problems for those inmates who came from urban areas. Because these urban males had "town fever in their veins," Hart judged that it was "practically impossible to keep them on farms" (p. 18). He explained that "home-sickness and distaste for farm labor attack many of them and they drift back sooner or later to city life" (p. 18). With regard to the "distaste for farm labor" that Hart had discerned, an accompanying photo under-scored his point. This photo, which is reproduced in Figure 4.1, was entitled "Learning to Be a Farmer." It revealed a smiling young male with a huge shovel. Readers did not require a great deal of imagination to infer the type of task in which this boy, who was standing in a pigsty, was about to engage.

Continued Support for Vocational Education

American vocational education expanded dramatically during the first quarter of the twentieth century. This growth, which was evident in special schools and asylums, was

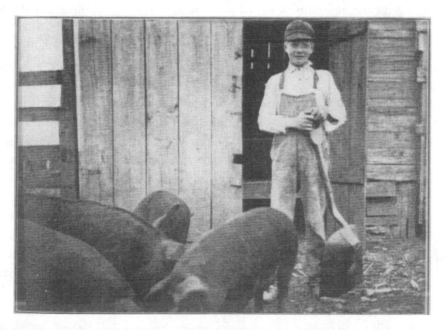

Figure 4.1. Early Twentieth-Century Photo Showcasing the Attractions of Farming.

inspired by European scholars. Lapage (1911), who was a British physician, had exhibited the attitudes of many European scholars. He had recommended that children with disabilities be exposed to academic studies. He believed that academics could be "an excellent means of providing training and employment for children without undue physical fatigue" (pp. 280–281). At the same time that he was endorsing academic activities, Lapage conceded that vocational activities also had value. He wrote that "work outside the school-room, physical labour [*sic*], is an equally good means of occupying and training those who are troublesome and robust" (p. 281).

Even though they were inspired by the Europeans, the American educators eventually did establish a distinctive philosophy. For example, William Holmes (1912) was a Rhode Island superintendent who disagreed with the pedagogical priorities that Lapage had set. Holmes believed that it was "the height of folly to try to teach [academic] studies to mentally defective children before they have had the preliminary work in sense training, muscular control, and manual work" (p. 81). He gave specific examples of the manual work that he had in mind. Holmes recommended "weaving, folding, cutting and bookbinding" for young males and females. He encouraged "mending, patching, and machine sewing" for older female students. Holmes encouraged older male students to "work at whittling, modeling, and benchwork [*sic*] in wood and iron" (p. 80). He added that children with disabilities "must be trained to habits of attention before they can take up with much success the more formal school work, such as reading, arithmetic and language" (p. 81).

Holmes was one of the many American special educators who debated about the relative importance of manual and academic learning. Annoyed at the extent to which this debate had been politicized, some special educators searched for a pragmatic way to combine the two approaches. Wallin (1914), who was a Pennsylvania professor, gave an example of an integrated approach. Wallin agreed with those scholars who thought that children with disabilities should learn from an academic curriculum. However, he thought that a vocational curriculum should be "provided for young adolescents (say, from twelve or thirteen to about sixteen years of age) who are appreciably backward or who are over age because of inability to cope with the regular curriculum, and who withal are industrially inclined" (p. 387). Even those students who had transferred to a vocation curriculum would continue to learn academic skills. Wallin explained that "the minimum of academic work provided should be closely correlated with the manual and industrial work" (p. 387).

Farrell (1914c) was the administrator in charge of special education for New York City. She quoted a section of a report that revealed the ways in which vocational education was being taught by New York City's special education teachers. Most of the teachers had been integrating vocational training with their academic instruction. Farrell recognized that the report's authors abhorred these practices.

> The usual program [in special education classes] is the three R's in the forenoon, and some form of handwork (manual training) in the afternoon. Nearly all of the experienced teachers and the principals are agreed that this bookwork is largely wasted upon these children; but they feel compelled to try to do this because it is the tradition of the system, and because the parents insist that their children shall be taught to read and write. (Passage from the *School Inquiry Report on Ungraded Classes*, 1912, as quoted by Farrell, 1914c, p. 99)

The authors of the preceding passage had firm convictions about vocational education. Those convictions should have been evident from the editorialized style of writing that they had employed. However, the authors decided to strengthen their stance on vocational training; they recommended that it become "the principal thing in all [special education] classes." As for academic learning, they suggested that "such reading, writing, and numbers as are taught should be taught, so far as possible, in connection with the hand work" (passage from the *School Inquiry Report on Ungraded Classes*, 1912, as quoted by Farrell, 1914c, p. 99).

Although Farrell (1914c) respectfully quoted advice from the *School Inquiry Report on Ungraded Classes*, she disagreed with that advice. She explained why she particularly resented the pragmatic approach that the report's authors had taken.

> Those who looked to the School Inquiry Investigation as the logical means of solving the problems now troubling school administrators in the fields of special education, [*sic*] will study the report in vain for a philosophy upon which to found their practice. . . . [That the authors of this report were] unable to see the forest for the trees is sad. To have missed the vision is sadder still. (p. 106)

The observations in the preceding paragraph were made by Farrell (1914c), who was the administrator in charge of special education for New York City. Anderson (1917) held a comparable administrative position in Newark, New Jersey. Anderson discouraged Newark's teachers from setting unrealistic goals for the students in their vocational education programs. She explained that "the feeble-minded will never enter the professions" nor would they "be trained to enter the skilled trades" (p. 82). Despite these cautions, Anderson felt that certain types of career training were suitable for persons with disabilities. She provided 16 examples.

1. Handy men around a place
2. Dish washers in hotels
3. Window cleaners for trolley or railroad companies
4. Assistant janitors
5. Cleaners in bakeries, butcher shops, etc.
6. Helpers for drivers on wagons
7. Domestic servants
8. Barbers' assistants
9. Laundry workers
10. Assistants to masons
11. Assistants to carpenters
12. Factory work which requires much repetition
13. Errand boys for tailors
14. Cobbling and shoe repairing
15. Bootblacks
16. Chair caners (pp. 82–83)

Anderson qualified the preceding list with a note that it was "probably incomplete."

Anderson (1917) had crafted a list of careers for male students. However, she also gave examples of occupations that were suitable for disabled female students. Some of these occupations involved needle work.

> Knitting and crocheting have proved most useful to many defective girls. . . . The defective girls will often knit and crochet during idle moments, and in that way are kept from associating with doubtful persons and getting into mischief. It is not claimed that knitting and crocheting are a panacea for immorality and mischief for defective girls; but if perhaps one, now and then, keeps herself busy and interested in her simple manual occupation, something, however little, has been accomplished. (p. 91)

School administrators established numerous special vocational education programs in the United States during World War I. Woodrow (1919) encapsulated the philosophy that undergirded most of these programs. He wrote that "all authorities" agreed that children with disabilities required "a more immediately practical education" (p. 259). Woodrow then explained that "the principle to follow is to teach only those things which the child can without doubt master sufficiently to make of them a real asset in such life work as he can be trained to do successfully" (pp. 259–260). The preparation for the "life-work which the child may ultimately make his own" required teachers to assess that child's "entire history, background and constitution" (p. 260). Woodrow made "a very conservative estimate" that more than 10 percent of the children in the schools would benefit from this type of special assessment and vocational training.

Although he was a strong advocate of vocational special education, Woodrow (1919) dutifully recapitulated the challenges that critics had made to this approach. However, he then attempted to answer these challenges. Two years earlier, Anderson (1917) also had recognized some of the shortcomings of vocational special education. Unlike Woodrow, Anderson sympathized with the critics. For example, she sided with those critics who had questioned whether "good training" could raise the job performance of persons with disabilities. Anderson pointed out that the data corroborating vocational training were "not sufficient to make one absolutely certain" (p. 83). Despite her reservations, Anderson professed that she had limited confidence in special vocational education. To help her readers understand the basis for that limited confidence, she provided them with two anecdotes. Both anecdotes were extremely macabre. Additionally, they both involved incidents that had transpired in the Newark school system, where Anderson worked as an administrator.

> The reports of cases of defective criminals show of what the untrained defective is capable. One boy killed his employer because he had asked him to do "things he didn't want to do." Another boy killed his teacher because under pressure from his parents she was trying to fit him for college when she should have been training him to do unskilled labor. These stories could be multiplied indefinitely. (pp. 84–85)

Like Anderson, Mead (1918) sympathized with the critics of special vocational education. Like Anderson, Mead based her opinion on anecdotal information. However, Mead relied on incidents that had transpired in Boston. She reported about the fates of 14 males and 4 females who had graduated from special education programs and then taken jobs in that community. Mead was disheartened that five of the boys, who had secured jobs as messengers, were employed for periods that lasted only several weeks. She noted that they "sickened of work" or were "thrown out for inefficiency" (p. 177). Four other lads, who were hired in shoe factories, quit because they were "desiring more pay" or "dissatisfied with work" (p. 178).

Mead (1918) recounted other incidents about students with disabilities. A disabled female who had been trained in the Boston schools was involved in one of these incidents. Mead thought this particular incident had revealed a problem with the "value" of the labor that the student had provided. Mead concluded that this young woman's problems generalized to other students with disabilities.

> Here is account of a girl now twenty-one, whose record in employment is as follows: during a period of two and half years, from sixteen to nineteen, she has occupied

eighteen different positions varying from nine days' to six months' service. . . . These facts are very significant and indicate, in the cases of girls, especially, maladjustment to the present conditions of employment and lack of proper supervision. (p. 179)

Special educators continued to argue about vocational training. Merrill (1918) was a Minnesota researcher who asked a question that was critical to this debate. After noting that many children could learn both academic and vocational skills, she asked "to what extent shall we emphasize the one [set of skills] at the expense of the other?" (p. 89). Merrill concluded that vocational skills should be emphasized. However, she warned the advocates of vocational education that the success of their approach would depend on whether it effectively prepared students "to meet the requirements of society or to contribute to their maintenance under supervision" (p. 89).

Advocates of vocational education recognized the complexity of the questions that educators were posing about vocational education. However, most of them also recognized the appropriateness of those questions. In an attempt to provide a convincing rejoinder, Bernstein (1918) made several observations about the New York asylum that he managed. He noted that he budgeted $48,000 annually so that his patients could operate a farm. After conceding that $48,000 constituted a significant amount of money, Bernstein pointed out that that the patients offset this cost by producing $90,000 worth of crops each year.

Porteus (1920), who was the director of research at the New Jersey training school in Vineland, realized that educators were frustrated by their inability to resolve some of the problems associated with student employment. He advised them to consider the full complexity of the problems that they were confronting. He also advised them that they should expect to remain frustrated until they accurately had assessed the entire range of potentially relevant variables. To help them make this assessment, he recommended that they compile student profiles. These profiles were to include measures of each student's general physical development, physiological brain capacity, psychological aptitude, educational ability, and temperament. Porteus then illustrated how these data could be collapsed into a composite index. The index would be coordinated with a vocational scale on which the relative difficulty of jobs had been identified. This vocational scale, which is illustrated in Figure 4.2, was intended to help the educators select the careers in which their students would succeed.

Spaulding (1920) recognized that that his fellow educators were having a difficult time ascertaining the optimal way to teach vocational skills to persons with disabilities. However, he thought this question was "not one of the more difficult questions" to resolve. Spaulding belittled their efforts, which he thought had focused on "the merely technical side of the vocation" (p. 75). Spaulding was more concerned about a closely connected "practical problem," namely "the development of vocational

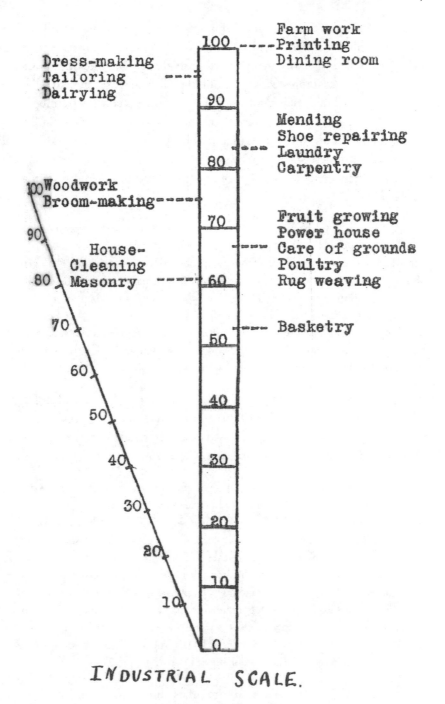

Figure 4.2. Early Twentieth-Century Scale Designed to Identify Careers for Special Learners.

or life intelligence, which is even more important than skill or semi-skill" (p. 75). Despite the cavalier manner in which he had assessed his antagonists' weaknesses, Spaulding had failed to clarify the practical problem to which he had alluded.

Gesell (1921) was impressed with Spaulding's line of reasoning. Gesell agreed that persons with disabilities would not benefit from technical training unless they possessed the intelligence to succeed at the career to which that training was linked. He alluded to the difficulties that disabled persons encountered when they were able to complete technical tasks but were not "able to save . . . or spend . . . with prudence" (p. 57). Gesell then proposed an ingenious solution for this problem.

> [Persons with disabilities] need vocational guidance in a very vigorous sense. They must not only be placed properly in an industry or an occupation, but they must be kept under a form of vocational probation and supervision. The goal should be to keep as many subnormal youths as possible in their local community, happy, secure, productive. This goal can be reached if we abandon the present practice of *laissez faire*, and substitute a sincere policy of after care, appointing an after care [*sic*] director to organize this important social service, and to secure the co-operation of parents, employers, and social welfare agencies in the solution of the problems. (Italics as in the original, p. 57)

The plan that Gesell proposed in 1921 already had been implemented in Boston during World War I. Fitts (1916; 1920), who was the supervisor in charge of that city's special education programs, had described details of this early program. She also had alluded to some of the reasons why the program was successful.

> The latest development in the organization of Special Classes is After-Care Work. About three years ago the Boston School Department assigned one Special Class teacher to follow-up the pupils after they had left the schools. . . . When a boy or girl reaches the age when he or she may legally leave school all assistance desired is given in finding suitable employment. This teacher guides them to lines of work for which they are adapted—and as far as possible steers them away from undesirable employment and blind alleys. She is known to many employers of unskilled labor who takes [*sic*] these Special Class pupils with full understanding of their limitations. She keeps track of them when they change employment and they come repeatedly for guidance and advice. . . . She is respected and consulted by the judges of juvenile courts where her following up leads her all too frequently. (Fitts, 1920, pp. 121–122)

Walter Fernald (1923) reviewed testimonials about the effectiveness of vocational education. On the basis of these endorsements, he concluded that "boys with nine or ten or eleven year mentalities who leave these classes should be able to go directly into industry and obtain good wages" (p. 405). Fernald was especially enthusiastic about community-based vocational training. He wrote that this geographically customized training would provide students with the skills that they needed to compete for distinctive employment opportunities in their own communities.

> The special training in these workshop classes should be varied according to the leading industries in the various cities. In the shoe city the handling of leather and the various work process making up the shoe industry should be taught in detail. In the textile city the spinning of yarns, the handling of cloth, etc., should be specifically taught. (p. 405)

Walter Fernald assured his readers that "the pupils who have done this sort of thing go back to these cities and get jobs without difficulty" (p. 405).

Descoeudres (1928) was a French educator who was committed to vocational education. Like Walter Fernald, she made suggestions about the best ways to organize vocational curricula. Some of her recommendations may have seemed odd to her tradition-minded colleagues in the United States.

> *Embroidery, sewing, crochet,* and *knitting,* which are confined to girls in the great majority of our schools, have already been introduced into boys' schools in several countries of Northern Europe, and also into most of our classes and institutions for defectives in Switzerland. In addition to the advantages of these occupations in the matter of manual skill a great service is done to the boys by making them capable of mending their own clothes in case of emergency. (Italics as in the original, p. 133)

Anticipating that some educators would question her advice, Descoeudres assured them that she had seen "backward boys learn to knit or sew much more rapidly than many normal girls" (p. 133).

During World War I, special educators had recommended a limited range of careers for students with disabilities. After the war, they continued to sanction only few types of employment. Taliaferro (1930) indicated that she had relied on the results of army testing data to discover those occupations that were appropriate for individuals with mental ages between 10 and 12. She thought that these persons could become artificial limb makers, asbestos workers, tent makers, or pastry cooks. She suggested that students with a mental age lower than 10 seek careers as bath attendants, hat renovators, tile setters, or window cleaners. After asserting that vocational programs could help students, Taliaferro added that they also could help parents. She noted that the parents could become "acquainted with the facts regarding the child's limitations, so that they may help plan the social and economic future" (p. 4). In view of the direct and indirect benefits of special vocational education, Taliaferro recommended wider implementation.

Summary

Asylums were seen as an effective ways to curb criminal activity, immoral conduct, and wanton propagation. Nonetheless, critics preferred community-based residences, which were less cruel and less expensive. They predicted that the patients at community-based homes would lead more satisfying lives. They predicted that some of them eventually would be able to live independently. They noted that the group homes, which were relatively inexpensive, could be managed even less expensively if the patients worked. In order to prepare patients for work, they turned to vocational training. They even persuaded public-school administrators to implement vocational training programs for students.

5

Political Liabilities and Opportunities

The history of the care and training of the handicapped must of necessity follow social and educational trends rather than create them [because] the wounded do not form the advance guard for an army.
—Trampton & Rowell, 1938

Some nineteenth-century reformers had depicted asylums as stark, restrictive, and expensive. They hoped that the public schools could serve as alternatives. They envisioned the schools as sites of programs that would develop general, academic, and vocational skills. They predicted that some of the participants in these programs would be able to procure jobs and live independently. They lobbied for legislation to advance their initiatives.

Politics in Europe

Most nineteenth-century Americans assumed that disabled persons posed a genuine threat to them. Several groups attempted to discredit this assumption. These groups included the families of disabled persons and humanitarian-minded citizens. They also included professionals, such as those educators and physicians who interacted with disabled persons. American scholars eventually joined this coalition. However, their European colleagues had pioneered the efforts to help persons with disabilities.

Franz (1912) was one of the many European scholars who had promoted an attitudinal shift toward persons with disabilities. When he later looked back on those early initiatives, Franz judged that he and his reform-minded associates had achieved many of the goals that they had set for themselves. He thought that they had been particularly successful in changing the attitudes of medical practitioners. Although he believed that the attitudes of numerous medical professionals with diverse specializations had changed, Franz concluded that in no branch had the prevailing "viewpoint more changed than in psychiatry" (p. 1).

Franz (1912) was aware that more and more groups were adopting new attitudes toward persons with disabilities. However, he believed that the new attitudes had historical roots. Franz noted that "the modern conception of insanity had its origin about a hundred years ago" (p. 1). This had been a period during which European scholars had "not only metaphorically but also actually, broke the chains that bound the insane" (p. 1). As a result of their sustained efforts, the early European scholars had been able to influence the attitudes of those professionals who had been providing healthcare. For example, they had had an impact on the directors of European hospitals and asylums. Franz believed that these directors had begun to view persons with disabilities differently. He judged that the directors had made "physical, mental and social treatment" the hallmarks of the programs at their institutions. To facilitate and accelerate institutional change, the directors had enlisted support from the families of patients, members of the general public, and government officials.

After he personally had assumed a new perspective toward mental disabilities, Franz (1912) encouraged his medical contemporaries to follow his example. Even though many practitioners did join him, Franz recognized that institutional changes would be expedited if they were associated with a political movement. The type of political movement that he had in mind required broad public support. Other professionals agreed with Franz. Therefore they invited the general public to join their discussions about disabled persons. During these discussions, Franz and the other professionals displayed remarkable rhetorical and political skills. However, some earlier advocates had demonstrated equally sophisticated skills.

Samuel Tuke

Although many nineteenth-century European scholars employed impressive political skills, the members of Great Britain's Tuke family stood out. Samuel Tuke (1815b) had been particularly prominent. Tuke, who was an influential European physician and educator, had tried to persuade professional colleagues and the public to treat persons with disabilities more humanely.

Recognizing that civic leaders and members of the public would reject any advice that seemed to imperil their safety, Samuel Tuke employed great tact. For example, he did not rail against restrictive facilities. Instead, he argued that restrictive facilities could be made to appear more hospitable. He wrote that "whatever lessens the prison-like appearance of these abodes, [sic] is deserving of attention" (p. 40). Samuel Tuke again displayed his rhetorical tact when he advised superintends to change the appearance of cast-iron window frames in British asylums. He thought that these frames should be replaced with ones that still were made of iron but that seemed to be made of wood. Tuke anticipated that critics would object that security was "an object to which even cheerfulness is but secondary" (1815b, p. 40). In complete agreement, he reassured them that window frames resembling wood were so secure that the "have been found entirely to supersede the necessity of iron grating" (p. 40).

Samuel Tuke (1815b) had made his remarks about the appearance of asylum windows in a manuscript that he wrote for medical personnel, civic leaders, and those architects who were designing asylums. Tuke showed political sophistication throughout this manuscript. Although he did lament the depressing environments in which persons with disabilities were housed, Tuke did not blame the architects.

> The construction of [the] Lunatic Asylum has, till of late years, occupied but little attention . . . and has displayed, if possible, still less ingenuity. The imperfection of these structures is not, however, altogether chargeable on the architectural profession.—One [sic] reason for their defects may be found in the rarity of such erections, which excited but little stimulus, and led few, if any, to study the wants of their inhabitants. Besides, it is the business of the architect to provide what is likely to be used; and it would have been a waste of talent to have devised the means for that discrimination, which was not employed in actual treatment. (pp. v–vi)

In the preceding passage, Tuke may have seemed excessively ingratiating to the architects. However, he recognized that the impact of his manuscript would have been reduced if it alienated one of the primary audiences for which it had been written.

Daniel Tuke

Daniel Tuke, who was the son of Samuel Tuke, was as politically sophisticated as his father. In an 1868 book, Daniel Tuke and a colleague (Bucknill & Tuke, 1968) used compliments rather than threats to change the attitudes of their readers. Directing their book chiefly at physicians, they assured them that "knowledge of the nature and treatment of Insanity [sic] is now expected of every well-educated medical man" and that the "desire to obtain a competent knowledge of this important branch of medical practice has become far more general in the profession than it ever before has been" (p. ix).

Daniel Tuke marketed later books in an equally clever fashion. He hoped that one of those books would persuade not only physicians but also "non-medical readers . . . to regard in a different light . . . the success of some of the fashionable modes of treatment" (1878, p. xi). Daniel Tuke specifically appealed to those members of the public who had turned to "modern spiritualism" to provide an explanation for mental disabilities. He urged the persons in this group to consult his book instead. When Daniel Tuke (1882) later wrote a history of disabilities in Great Britain, he stated that "every friend of humanity ought to be acquainted" with his volume.

In multiple instances, Daniel Tuke used flattery to change the attitudes of the public. However, he also employed negative strategies. Possibly disappointed that more persons had not purchased his earlier materials, he began one of his last books by chastising members of the public. He scolded them for "the languid interest now felt in the stirring events" that he was recounting in his book. This lack of interest "by the general public, and even many medical men," struck Tuke as "not a little surprising, seeing that one in every three hundred of the population suffers from mental disorder and has good reason to be thankful that he is not lying in a dark cell on straw, 'being bound in affliction and iron' " (1892c, p. 2).

Daniel Tuke (1878) had explicitly discussed the influence of politics on the ways that American citizens treated disabled persons. He was particularly fascinated with those physicians who had concluded that America's political culture was in some peculiar fashion a cause of disabilities. Daniel Tuke explained that "in America, medical men have for many years . . . protested against the evil influences at work in their social and the political life" (p. 196). He recapitulated additional allegations.

> [One physician] thought that . . . evils were but too plainly exemplified in the mental traits characteristic of "young America," [sic] and in the increasing stream of depravity, and disease both physical and mental, which permeated the social fabric, and threatened to injure not only the present but future generations. Another finds a cause of insanity in the neglect and misdirection of early education, and inveighs strongly against the excessive freedom of thought and action exercised by every individual; the high degree of excitement called forth in the pursuits of life; emulation; the rapid succession of sorrow, and joy, fear, and hope, and consequent loss of mental equilibrium. (p. 197)

Tuke approvingly quoted an American physician who had noted that the American "form of government, with the habits of our people, is calculated to increase rather than diminish the frequency of insanity" (Anonymous American physician, n.d., as quoted by Tuke, 1878, pp. 197–198).

Like many of his contemporaries, Daniel Tuke was aware of the degree to which the attitudes of professionals influenced the public's attitudes toward persons with disabilities. He also realized that these attitudes influenced the government officials who established policies, managed practices, and allocated funding. Because he was politically astute, Tuke attempted to not only navigate but control the contemporary political currents. Nonetheless, he may have underestimated the extent to which he was controlled by the same forces that he hoped to regulate. The influence of these forces may have been apparent in the haughty remarks that Tuke had made about the Americans. It was revealed again when he discussed the changing social behaviors of patients. He wrote that "disregard for external appearance" was a "frequent indication of incipient insanity" (1878, p. 216). To make sure that his readers did not misunderstand him, Tuke instructed them to be on the alert for the instance in which "a man who was tidy in his habits before, [*sic*] becomes slovenly and careless in his dress" (p. 216).

Daniel Tuke had believed that certain behaviors indicated mental disabilities. However, the significance of these behaviors had been controversial even during the late 1800s. The extent of this controversy was revealed in one of his highly politicized reports. In that report, Daniel Tuke (1878) addressed the legal liability that physicians incurred when they attempted to institutionalize patients against their wishes. In fact, he recounted details of cases in which indignant patients had won judgments against the doctors. Daniel Tuke concentrated his attention upon a particular case in which the judge had reached a conclusion that Tuke personally endorsed. He noted that this judge "happily availed himself of pointing out to the legislature the necessity for there being clauses in any Lunacy Bill" to protect physicians from "unjustifiable" legal actions (p. 10). Daniel Tuke proclaimed that "the importance of the result of this case can scarcely be over-estimated" (p. 10).

John Batty Tuke

John Batty Tuke was another member of that illustrious family within Great Britain's special education establishment. John Batty Tuke was a distinguished physician, the medical superintendent at a Scottish asylum, and a leader among those professionals who wished to improve the lives of disabled individuals. Because he was a citizen in a country in which social and educational experiments were being conducted, John Batty Tuke had the opportunity to gauge the reactions of his countrymen to these pioneering initiatives. He may have been especially concerned about the many initiatives that had been championed by members of his own family.

Like Samuel Tuke and Daniel Tuke, John Batty Tuke did not ignore those members of the public who were fearful of persons with disabilities. In fact, he specifically acknowledged that "great anxiety is already felt in many of the districts of

Scotland at the gradually increasing number of pauper lunatics" (John Batty Tuke, 1868, p. 916). After he had noted that citizens were reluctant to allow this epidemic to continue, Tuke added that even "greater reluctance is evidenced on the part of the ratepayers to increase asylum accommodation" (p. 916). Simultaneously concerned about their own safety and the high cost of institutionalization, the Scottish citizens had begun to experiment with less expensive facilities, such as group homes. The Scotts eventually concluded that the group homes were safe as well as affordable. John Batty Tuke paraphrased their conclusion, which was that the communal living model "for harmless lunatics and idiots provides amply against any further expenditure in adding to the Royal and District Asylums" (p. 916).

John Batty Tuke had made the preceding comments in 1863. Thirty-five years later, he had been appointed as a Lecturer on Insanity at the School of Medicine of the Royal Colleges at Edinburgh. He also had been designated President of Scotland's Royal College of Physicians. John Batty Tuke used his professional prominence as the vantage from which to fire a broadside at some of Great Britain's current social policies. John Batty Tuke was sure that these policies had created many dysfunctional political situations.

> During the . . . last century vast changes were brought about in the principles governing the management of the insane in France and Great Britain, and . . . it has been deemed desirable to commemorate the centenary of a beneficent revolution. But I doubt much whether this epochal consideration has had much to do with the matter; more do I think that the request of [the British Medical Association] for addresses on the subject have been prompted by social considerations affection the general public. Doubtless the rapidly-increasing [*sic*] incubus of lunacy is seriously complicating Poor-law administration, but the question of relief from its pressure is not one that can be referred to the opinion of a single individual. (Tuke, 1898, p. 341)

John Batty Tuke (1898) made the preceding remarks as part of an address to the British Medical Association. Instead of simply criticizing the treatment and education of persons with disabilities, he could have used this address to provide advice about ways to improve the current system. However, John Batty Tuke recommended that this advice be solicited from a special commission that was to be appointed for this precise purpose. The commission that he had in mind would consist "of authorities in lunacy, representative from the general profession, lawyers, and Poor-law administrators" (p. 341). John Batty Tuke argued that the suggestions of this politically stratified group "might influence future policy and arrest the haphazard drifting one which at present obtains" (p. 341).

William Ireland

William Ireland (1877) was a British scholar who had written an influential book about the distinctive pedagogical practices that special educators should employ. Near the end of the nineteenth century, Ireland (1898) wrote another significant book, which he entitled *The Mental Affections of Children, Idiocy, Imbecility and Insanity*. In the preface to this latter volume, Ireland indicated that he wished to influence a general audience as well as a professional one. Ireland explained his hope "that some parts of [this book] will be found . . . useful to those who have the care and guardianship of idiots and imbeciles, or who take a philanthropic interest in provisions for their welfare" (p. v).

In order to lure general readers to his 1898 book, Ireland appealed directly to them. However, he and his publisher then took their marketing plan a step further. They strategically assembled a 12-page supplement that contained reviewers of Ireland's previous works. Within these promotional excerpts, the reviewers had indicated that general audiences should read Ireland's books. Ireland's publisher used these reviews as an appendix in Ireland's new book.

Politics in Nineteenth-Century America

Zedler (1953) acknowledged the ways in which the American debate about children with disabilities had changed during the nineteenth and twentieth centuries. Looking back on the preceding 75 years, he concluded that the "policies affecting the attendance of [children with disabilities] in public schools have been the direct outgrowth of 'play of public opinion and the political complex of pressure and agitation'" (p. 187). Zedler reasoned that the proponents of change were successful largely because of the political pressure that they had exerted on the "the administrative, legislative and judicial organs of government" (p. 187). Medical and educational leaders had helped apply the political pressure to which Zedler had referred. They had developed that pressure while they were addressing parents, guardians, managers of asylums, and school administrators. They also created it while they were interacting with community leaders and government officials.

Some of the events in nineteenth-century Massachusetts illustrated the type of political dynamics to which Zedler (1953) had referred. The Massachusetts citizens had been extremely progressive in the way that they had established and regulated special education. Their attitudes had been evident in some of the actions that they had taken in the middle of the nineteenth century. For example, the 1846 Massachusetts legislature had appointed a commission to determine an appropriate means of caring for mentally disabled persons. To discharge their task, the members of this commission decided to establish an experimental facility. Although he agreed with this plan, Howe advised the other commission members to delay construction. He thought that they first should identify the number of persons in Massachusetts who would be eligible for admission to this type of facility. Therefore, Howe and several colleagues began to visit the cities, towns, and villages of Massachusetts in order to count the numbers of disabled persons at each stop. After they had completed this task, Howe summarized their findings. In an 1848 report, he documented that "five hundred and seventy-four [disabled] human beings" lived in those towns where he had stopped. He noted that the persons in question were individuals "who are condemned to hopeless idiocy, who are considered and treated as idiots by their neighbors, and left to their own brutishness" (Howe, 1972, p. viii). Howe judged that all of these persons would have been eligible for admission to the new facility. By extrapolating from the samples in the towns and cities that he had visited, he estimated that 1500 state residents would qualify for admission to the Massachusetts facility.

The Massachusetts commission eventually did develop an experimental facility. Howe (1851) anticipated some of the reactions that persons would exhibit after they had visited the new facility. He predicted that most visitors "would find it hard to say a word of approval or encouragement" (p. 102). Howe felt that these negative impressions would be the result of misunderstandings. Even though the current conditions may have seemed deplorable, Howe believed that they were superior to the prior conditions in which the patients had lived. Additionally, he though that the patients at the Massachusetts facility had made genuine progress. Howe advised potential visitors, as well as the legislators who had funded the project that the patients' current "condition furnishes a fair specimen of what may become the condition of all, if the State will take [additional persons with mental disabilities] under her fostering care" (p. 103).

Ray (1852) was another Massachusetts physician who wished to help persons with disabilities. Although he was an advocate of asylums, Ray agreed with Howe that visitors had formed negative impressions of the asylums. In fact, Ray identified some of the specific allegations that visitors had made about a Massachusetts asylum.

> It is supposed that patients are not treated with invariable kindness; that the management is harsh and cruel; that obedience is enforced by blows or rough handling; that refractory conduct is met by the discipline of shower-baths or confinement in dark dungeons; that they are neglected when sick; that they have improper and insufficient food; that their friends are not allowed to visit them; and finally, that to favour [*sic*] the schemes of interested relatives, persons are deprived of their liberty under a mere pretence of insanity. (p. 38)

Wishing to dispel these perceptions, Ray suggested that "the most prolific source of this distrust . . . is, undoubtedly, the communication of patients themselves, the more effective for falling, as they generally do, on willing ears" (pp. 38–39). Ray adjured members of the public to ignore their relatives and place their trust in the administrators at asylums.

Although some physicians, special educators, and members the public were interested in the conditions of patients at asylums, most of them were more concerned about the ways in which disabled persons could damage society. Jarvis (1852), a Massachusetts physician, identified a British scholar who had explained the basis for the prevailing fear of disabled persons. This scholar had maintained that "a very general apprehension has existed both in this country and France, that Insanity [sic] has increased in prevalence of late years, to an alarming extent, and that the number of lunatics, when compared with the population, is continually on the increase" (J. C. Prichard, n.d., as quoted by Jarvis, 1852, p. 333). Jarvis added his own opinion that "a very similar apprehension exists in America" (1852, p. 333). Jarvis then cited data to "corroborate the opinion of nearly all writers, whether founded on positive and known facts, on analogy, on computation or on conjecture, that insanity is an increasing disease" (p. 364).

Toward the end of the nineteenth century, Warner (1894) observed that government-based services for persons with disabilities had passed through three distinct stages. In the initial stage, the government had provided educational services only to "the deaf, the dumb, and the blind." In the intermediate stage, the government had helped "the insane" find accommodations within hospitals or asylums. However, Warner believed that the efforts made during the intermediate stage had languished because of "the great expense of providing for the increasing numbers of the chronic insane" (p. 142). In the last stage, the government had established "educational institutions for the feeble-minded" (p. 142). Warner acknowledged that the last stage of development had "only recently made much headway."

Assigning Political Responsibility for Disabilities

Some members of the public acknowledged a political responsibility to help disabled persons. They then had a choice of personally accepting that responsibility or assigning it to someone else. Most persons preferred to delegate it. The manner in which the public delegated this responsibility was entwined with its perceptions about which group was to blame for disabilities. Seguin (1870), an influential French educator who had relocated to the United States, attempted to direct the blame away from handicapped children. However, he did this in a way that had clear political implications. Seguin's political intentions were evident when he melodramatically identified some of the incidental circumstances that could contribute to disabilities.

> I have attended a mother of a remarkably fine family of four children, whose fifth was affected. . . . During that pregnancy, her husband was deeply involved in speculations; he would say nothing to her about his chances, but she knew daily, the way he ate, how much he had lost. One day she saw him swallow his dinner without masticating at all; she fainted away, the child hardly moved after, and was born a cripple and an idiot. (p. 31)

It was unlikely that readers would fail to comprehend the moral of the preceding story. Nonetheless, Seguin (1870) reinforced that message. He advised women "who would cherish the idea of raising a brood of loving creatures" to marry poor but fiscally responsible cobblers. Seguin adjured the women to turn down any suitor who had "a suspicious bank-book" or who aspired to own a "mortgaged high-stoop residence" (p. 31). As a final caveat, Seguin observed that "man suffers through his head and heart" but that "woman suffers besides, and more, through her womb" (p. 32).

Seguin (1870) had directed many of his remarks at those individuals who had treated disabled persons harshly. Like Seguin, Kerlin (1885) disapproved of those individuals who wished to discipline or punish disabled persons. He especially resented those members of the public who wished to kill persons with disabilities. Kerlin wrote that the political extremists who favored "extinction" had forgotten "how far such practice would be from all moral or judicial right, how revolting to every religious sentiment and contradictory to every logical principle" (p. 249). Kerwin noted that the zealots had erred by focusing their attention exclusively on the "preservation of society itself from a baneful, hindering, or disturbing element" (p. 249). As a result, they had failed to consider a fundamental right of every disabled person. Kerlin expressed this as the right "inherently existing in a defective and irresponsible member of society to protection from the body in exact ratio to his necessities" (p. 249). Kerlin encouraged politically progressive government officials to replace "survival of the fittest" attitudes with "paternal" attitudes.

Barrows (1888) was another nineteenth-century scholar who was upset by extremists. To help readers understand the basis for his feelings, Barrows described a distressing encounter with a fellow Massachusetts resident. Barrows characterized this resident as "a very intelligent man, a graduate of Harvard University" (p. 396).

> I said to him: "Doctor, what shall be done with this problem of the feeble-minded? There are seventy-six thousand of them in the United States alone." He

had a solution ready. It is a solution you have heard of before. . . . He said, "I would stamp out and kill off the whole brood." (p. 396)

The nineteenth-century extremists who favored harsh treatments were not intimidated by the rhetoric of Barrows (1888) and other reformers. Writing originally in 1893, Henderson (1901), who was a professor at the University of Chicago, dismissed the reformers as idealists who had underestimated the "moral insensibility" of persons with disabilities. To clarify his notion of moral insensibility, Henderson explained that "a slight lapse of truth will give a morally healthy persons more bitter pangs of remorse than a murder accompanied by torture gives to most murderers" (p. 132). In contrast, Henderson believed that "in their cells criminals enjoy dreamless sleep and excellent appetite" and that "the only shame they feel . . . arises when the police have outwitted them" (p. 132). Equating disabled persons with criminals, Henderson asserted that they were members of "the human classes of arrested or perverted development who lie in the dark pool at the foot of our social ascent" (p. 138).

Like Henderson and other extremists, Alexander Johnson (1898) opposed the social reformers who were advocating special education. He judged that only "a few among the more advanced students of penology" had studied the criminal habits of persons with disabilities. Counting himself among those advanced students, Johnson concluded that disabled persons were habitual criminals who were "unfit for free, social life" (p. 326). He recommended that they be "debarred from pleasures and opportunities which they cannot or will not enjoy without injury to themselves and others" (p. 326). Johnson added that disabled persons "should, by all means, be prevented from leaving offspring who would probably inherit the evil tendencies of their parents" (p. 326). Johnson was particularly disconcerted that his opponents had begun to vilify him as a "political enthusiast."

At the end of the nineteenth century, the legislators of Massachusetts had become famous for implementing politically progressive programs. In spite of this enviable reputation, some government leaders in Massachusetts were unsympathetic to these progressive initiatives that benefited persons with disabilities. Rogers (1898) documented the caustic remarks of Governor Butler during his 1883 address to the Massachusetts Legislature. Governor Butler observed that "it will be time enough to undertake the education of the idiotic and the feeble-minded" after Massachusetts "shall have sufficiently educated every bright child within its borders" (Governor Butler, 1883, as quoted by Rogers, 1898, p. 152). Governor Butler added that the prerequisite funding for special education was unavailable. However, he added that, even were that funding to become available, he would continue to oppose special education.

[Children with disabilities] in whom some spark of intelligence has been awakened, [*sic*] have become so ashamed of their school that when they write to their parents they beg for paper and envelopes which have not its card upon it. That is, they have been educated simply enough to know of their deficiencies and be ashamed of themselves and their surroundings. We do not contribute to their happiness by giving them that degree of knowledge. (Governor Butler, 1883, as quoted by Rogers, 1898, pp. 152–153.)

Governor Butler concluded that "a well-fed, well-cared-for idiot, is a happy creature," while "an idiot awakened to his condition is a miserable one" (Governor Butler, 1883, as quoted by Rogers, 1898, p. 153).

Carson (1899), who was the superintendent of a New York asylum, had chaired a committee of the National Conference of Charities and Correction. Carson and the members of his committee had deliberated about some of the issues surrounding special education. Carson dutifully reported about Edward Seguin, the famous French educator, who claimed that the students in special education classes had been remarkably successful. However, Carson questioned the validity of Seguin's claims. He insisted that the number of persons with disabilities who were "advanced to a condition of normal intelligence and citizenship is extremely limited, if there are any at all" (p. 295). After writing alliteratively that Seguin had been too sanguine, Carson advised state legislators to ignore the French scholar's advice. Instead, they were to concentrate on enacting laws that would protect society. Carson and the members of his committee explicitly backed laws "prescribing some extraordinary penalty . . . for the seduction of any insane, epileptic, or feeble-minded woman" (p. 303). They also endorsed laws that would prevent disabled persons from marrying.

When educators and politicians recommended harsh treatments, the parents of disabled youngsters objected. In most late nineteenth-century American communities, the parents only had two opportunities to educate children with disabilities. They could keep their children at home or send them away to an institution. Even if parents wished to educate their children at home, many of them lacked the skills, time, and resources. As for sending their children to an asylum, they had a difficult time locating one that was not overcrowded. If the parents could locate an asylum that was still accepting patients, they may have been distressed by the impersonal, repressive, or punitive treatments at the facility. Kerlin (1877), who objected to the negative fashion in which asylums were being characterized, reassured parents that "in the great majority of instances, [children with disabilities] are better and more successfully treated in well-organized institutions than is possible at their homes" (p. 21). Despite declarations of this sort from the directors of asylums, many parents suspected that conditions in the institutions were deplorable.

For both humane and practical reasons, more and more members of the public wished to find alternatives to asylums. Davies (1923) recognized that this political movement was gaining the attention of government officials and leaders. He referred to the era during which this movement began as "the modern period" of special education. Davies explained that this period was characterized by efforts to deal "with the large numbers of mental defectives in the population" by means of "extra-institutional methods of care, training and supervision" (p. 19). Community homes represented one of the "extra-institutional methods of care" to which Davies had referred. Residential schools, day-care facilities, and vocational training programs comprised other options.

Early in the twentieth century, Davies (1923) had made remarks about the political complexity of special education. However, some nineteenth-century educators had anticipated his remarks. For example, Powell (1887) had been aware of these political dynamics when he had attempted to explain the emergence of facilities for children and adults with disabilities. Powel initially had presented an idealized and simplistic rationale for these events. He stated that during the first quarter of the nineteenth century, "the leaven of Christian philanthropy lifted the environing prejudice of . . . darkened minds; and from this time on both public and private schools began to be established in Europe and America" (p. 251). Powell had made these remarks to the National Conference of Charities and Correction. Despite the simplicity of the preceding explanation, Powell was politically sophisticated at other times. He showed keen insight when he addressed the identical issue in a different section of his speech. In that separate section, Powell observed that the public actually had two reasons for "extending her mantle of charity to . . . the lowest and most helpless of mankind" (p. 259). One reason was indeed the "aiding and protecting [of] suffering humanity" (p. 259). However, the second reason, which was preeminently pragmatic, was to relieve "the community of an exhausting burden that in many families is overtaxing the parents and preventing prosperity and care of other members of the family" (p. 259).

Late Nineteenth-Century America Legislation

The different ways in which civic leaders viewed the origin of disabilities influenced the ways in which they crafted regional laws. Writing at the end of the nineteenth century, Randall (1896) reported about those Michigan legislators who had authorized special educational services in 1871. He indicated that they had modeled their initiative after one in France, where school administrators had established special education at the beginning of the nineteenth century. Prior to 1871, Michigan's legislators had relegated disabled children to county poorhouses. They eventually provided funding to the poorhouses in return for these extraordinary services. The Michigan legislators also had sent children to church-based asylums. As they had done with the poorhouses, they defrayed a portion of this care's cost. However, Randall discouraged legislators from continuing these practices. He believed that church-based facilities that received tax revenues had ceased to be charitable institutions. Randall wrote that they had turned into institutions that were "conducted by private parties for their own interest and seldom controlled by law as to admissions or discharges of children" (p. 712).

New York lawmakers passed legislation similar to that which their Michigan colleagues had implemented. Millis (1898) noted that New Yorkers previously had left disabled children with their parents, sent them to almshouses, or assigned them to "adults in the country." He observed that in 1875 New York legislators authorized the use of public funds to support children in church-based asylums. However, Millis judged that "this subsidy system [had] led to great abuses" (p. 777). Even though he recognized that financial abuses had occurred, Millis thought that private asylums remained valuable components of a comprehensive system of state care. He approvingly pointed to West Virginia and South Dakota, where lawmakers had authorized "the courts to commit dependent and vagrant children to societies to be placed out" (p. 779). Millis concluded that private asylums had evolved into "an important part of the system of almost every state" (p. 777).

In his report about state laws that were affecting persons with disabilities, Millis (1898) had reinforced the points that many of his contemporaries had been making. For example, he agreed with those persons who had applauded legislators for enacting laws to ensure that the "deaf and dumb and the blind" would be educated. At the same time, Millis chastised legislators for ignoring the educational interests of children with mental disabilities. Other scholars, such as Best (1930), would restate the point that Millis had made. Looking back on the period that Millis had studied, Best noted the different manners in which children with distinct types of disabilities had been treated. Best explained that "the work for the deaf and the blind proceeded apace till in time every state in the Union was providing for them, either in an institution within its borders or in one without" (p. 633). In contrast, "the work for the feeble-minded . . . soon slackened" (Best, 1930, p. 633). To substantiate this allegation, Best noted an historical dearth of state laws defining the rights of persons with mental disabilities. He reported that the type of legislation to which he was referring initially "did not make a place for itself in the organic law of the several states" (p. 633). Although Best alluded to several extenuating factors that had restricted the passage of such laws, he concluded that "the actual expense involved, when there were other and apparently more immediate calls on the public treasury to be attended to, was doubtless the prevailing cause for the circumscription of the work for the feeble-minded" (p. 634).

Most late nineteenth-century scholars recognized that ulterior political forces were influencing the course of special education. However, they adopted diverse philosophical perspectives from which to view these influences. After conducting a review of the programs that had been serving children with disabilities for the preceding 40 years, Wilbur (1888) concluded that these programs had emerged because the American public had demonstrated a broad commitment to special education. He observed that "the interest awakened in this country in this work is growing daily" (p. 111). However, Wilbur also believed that the politicians who had been committed to special education should receive some credit. He explained that "even 'reform politicians' are open to conviction concerning the necessity and economy of making reasonable provision" for disabled persons. Wilbur pointed to recent events in Nebraska to substantiate this view. He characterized Nebraska as a state that had "made liberal appropriations for establishing its institutions for the feeble-minded upon a basis commensurate with the wants and needs of its people" (p. 112).

Like Wilbur, Brown (1889) was another late nineteenth-century observer who was sure that ulterior political forces had influenced the course of special education. Like Wilbur, Brown encouraged her readers to applaud those government leaders who had shown an interest in special education. She explained that "it must be an axiomatic proposition that the State should educate all its dependent children" (p. 86). Brown believed that this mandate included children with disabilities, whom government leaders had "to educate like others, so far as possible" (p. 86).

Brown (1889) anticipated that citizens who agreed with her philosophical arguments still might object to special education because of the expenses that it entailed. However, she had prepared a retort. Brown observed that "I can see no reason why the means for such education should not be appropriated from the general school fund" (p. 86). She thought that this means of funding might be especially fitting because it would be a way of "providing for those of [a state's] own household, as when it furnishes schools for the well-endowed" (p. 86). Still worried that she might not have made her case in the most convincing fashion, Brown provided one more piece of macabre but persuasive information. She informed her readers that the cost of educating children with disabilities always would remain relatively modest because the children's "duration of life is somewhat less than for the well-endowed" (p. 88).

Salisbury (1892) was a nineteenth-century scholar who agreed that ulterior political forces were influencing the course of special education. However, he assumed a distinct perspective on those forces. Salisbury assigned a high priority to government leaders, whom he thought had a genuine responsibility to educate children with disabilities. Rather than linking this responsibility to some "axiomatic proposition," Salisbury rationalized it with a five-part argument. His argument blended theoretical, practical, and legal considerations.

1.   The State should systematically care for and train its feebleminded for the same reason that it educates its deaf and blind youth. . . .
2.   The State should nurture its feebleminded for the same reasons which demand the care of its insane. . . .
3.   The State should hasten to care for its feebleminded as a measure of social self-preservation, for the greater health, physical and moral, of the body social. . . .
4.   The State should guard and educate its feebleminded because this will never be done otherwise. . . .
5.   Last but not least, this thing should be done because it is unjust and unwise to discriminate against a single defective and unfortunate class. (pp. 229–231)

After he had developed this multifaceted argument, Salisbury published it so that his professional colleagues could read it. He also presented it to the state leaders of Wisconsin. He hoped that these state leaders would make his argument the foundation for progressive programs.

State legislators constituted only one of the groups that deliberated about nineteenth-century education. However, the legislators, who controlled funding, were important participants. Walter Fernald (1893), who was a Massachusetts school administrator, understood the power that legislators wielded. After identifying the states that initially had established educational institutions for children with disabilities, he noted that "nearly every one of these early institutions was opened at or near the capitals of their various States, [*sic*] in order that the members of the legislature might closely watch their operations" (p. 209). He urged school administrators to maintain the confidence of their legislators. Fernald also warned them that some of the legislators who once had supported special education had started to question its value. He reassured these legislators that "it is better and cheaper for the community to assume the permanent care of this class before they have carried out a long career of expensive crime" (p. 211). Fernald warned any legislators who were thinking of withdrawing their support that they should be prepared "to take charge of adult idiots in almshouses and hospitals, and of imbecile criminals in jails and prisons" (p. 211).

Political Changes in America During the Early 1900s

During the nineteenth century, members of public began to change their attitudes toward learners with disabilities. Throughout the early years of the twentieth century, they continued to adapt their attitudes. Their concerns about children with disabilities correlated with their concerns about several other important issues. For example, they correlated with their concerns about race. They also correlated with their concerns about economics, crime, and morality. As a consequence, these related issues influenced the public's attitudes toward learners with disabilities.

Exposure to skillful rhetoric was still another factor that influenced the public's attitudes toward learners with disabilities. Writing in the middle of the nineteenth century, Howe (1852) had demonstrated impressive rhetorical skills. Howe initially agreed with the critics of special education that "the degree in which [persons with disabilities] possess mind and knowledge varies . . . some having so little that they can hardly be distinguished from monkeys" (p. 9). After he had conceded this point, Howe immediately added that other persons with disabilities had so much mind and knowledge "that they can hardly be distinguished from other men" (p. 9).

Writing almost half a century after Howe, Lawrence (1900) rephrased Howe's basic argument in a manner that was even more persuasive.

> Feeble-mindedness is not an absolute state or condition. I mean to say that the line between feeble-mindedness and normal-mindedness is not a fixed affair; that feeble-mindedness is a relative state or condition; that there is as much difference between two feeble-minded children as there is between two children in the grades. . . . Now, in order to become interested in the personality of any one of these children, you must see and know the child. (p. 100)

Impressed by the reasoning of Lawrence and like-minded colleagues, more and more educators began to depict disabilities as points on a continuum that included normal as well as abnormal behaviors. For example, Burk (1900) pointed out that "there are so many and such varying conditions in the make-up of individual children that those differing from the normal will often be more in evidence than those approaching the normal" (p. 302). To resolve the ensuing problems, Burk suggested that teachers allow "each child the right to traverse the present curriculum at a pace which is normal to himself" (p. 302). The members of the National Education Association adopted an expansive pedagogical philosophy that was comparable to that which Burk had articulated. Their philosophy was to some degree evident in the inclusive name that they selected for their organization's new special education unit. They chose the extremely broad subtitle, *Department for Children Demanding Special Means of Instruction* (Bell, 1902, as quoted by Frampton & Gall, 1955a, p. 11).

The members of the National Education Association formally had decided to embrace special education at their 1902 convention. Writing several years later, Allen (1904), who was the principal at a Pennsylvania school for children with disabilities, reminisced about this decision. He also corroborated its importance. Allen wrote that "it is being more and more recognized that the line between a defective and a normal child cannot be drawn hard and fast, and that many a child who appears dull and stupid in school is in some measure defective" (p. 773). Allen judged that the impact of this "very recent movement" had been increased by the alliance between "the educators of the defective classes with those of the national educational association [*sic*]" (p. 773).

G. Stanley Hall was one of the most popular and influential psychologists at the beginning of the twentieth century. In remarks that he had made originally in 1901, Hall (1914) had predicted the increasing popularity of the relativist perspective on disability and individualized learning. He wrote that the concepts associated with this emerging perspective had become "basal for the new education." He predicted that "their far-off fruitage will be seen in more completely developed and more diversified personalities" (p. xix). He also predicted that leaders from the "home, church, and state" would collaborate to develop "broader conceptions of what education means" (p. xix).

Chace (1903) was sympathetic to Hall's 1901 remarks. She was a scholar who was distressed by the negative ways in which children with disabilities had been depicted. Chace particularly resented the professionals and members of the public who had associated special learners with traits such as "indolence or laziness." She assured her readers that disabled learners could be transformed into "self-respecting and self-supporting men and women" (p. 385). Exposing the learners to individualized educational programs was a critical step in this transformational process. Chace advised her readers that they had no choice but to educate all children with disabilities because those learners who were not educated "would degenerate into the ranks of the defectives and the delinquents" (p. 385).

Impetus for Public Special Education

Richman (1907), who was the superintendent of the New York City schools, was inspired by the recent progress that special educators had made in the public schools. This progress convinced him that the American educational system was benefiting from "a greater intelligence, a broader influence, and a sense of higher obligation" (p. 233). Even though he recognized the contributions that special educators were making, Richman still chastised them. He was particularly distressed by the manner in which they had concentrated their attention on children with physical disabilities. He believed that they had made this emphasis at the expense of children with mental disabilities. To clarify his point, Richman described a hypothetical group of 50 children. He pointed out that the students in such a group would "show almost fifty differences in height, weight and physical endurance" and that they would reveal "similar differences in the quality and quantity of brain power" (p. 233). Richman concluded that only individualized lessons could meet the mental needs of such a group.

Smart (1908) was another educator who wished to convince her readers that special education was valuable. Because she was convinced that educators were employing imprecise identification techniques, Smart assumed that any group of special learners would include some students who exhibited only borderline problems. However, Smart was not distressed by this situation. In fact, she tried to demonstrate that special education assisted students without genuine disabilities. To buttress her case, she quoted remarks from a fellow educator. This colleague had asserted that "one of the largest benefits that can be derived from allowing special children to work with the normal children in the public schools is the benefit that comes to us members of the normal community" (Marian Campbell, 1908, as quoted by Smart, 1908, p. 1151). Worrying that these corroborative comments could be misinterpreted as "a very selfish thing to say," Smart pointed to a particularly important way in which special education benefited "normal" learners. She indicated that it helped them develop a wholesome perspective toward their disabled classmates.

Advocates of special education presented multiple arguments to their professional colleagues and the public. For example, they depicted special education as a pragmatic and affordable way to protect society. Johnstone (1908) wrote that "we must use every endeavor in our special-class work to remove from the grades all children who physical or mental infirmities unfit [*sic*] them for normal life and progress with normal children" (p. 1115). Johnstone underscored the point that "it is the normal child who suffers most from contact with the special child who is unable to follow the work of the class" (p. 1115).

Johnstone (1908) had maintained that special education programs were worthwhile because they separated children with disabilities from the rest of the community. However, he pointed to an additional advantage: many of the learning techniques that had been devised originally in special classrooms could be extrapolated to regular education classrooms. To reinforce this point, Johnstone identified an operational principle from industry that he thought was appropriate for education.

> Just as in the great manufacturing industries, those things which were once thrown away as waste have become the most valuable output as by-products, so the incidental things in connection with the training of special children will, I believe, be the most important. (p. 1115)

Although the preceding observation may have been based on common business practices, it must have struck many parents as inappropriate.

Farrell (1908–1909), who had helped establish special education classes in New York City, did not restrict these innovative programs to children with disabilities. In fact, she admitted that she and her colleagues initially had downplayed the ways in which special educational programs benefited children with disabilities. Like other politically savvy teachers, she suggested that special educational programs were worthwhile because of the service that they provided to the entire community. Using New York City as an example, she reminisced that the programs originally "grew out of conditions in a neighborhood which furnished many and serious problems in truancy and discipline" (p. 91). Concerned about these problems, the local school administrators had established special education programs to accommodate not only children with disabilities but also "over-age children, so-called naughty children and the dull and stupid children" (p. 91).

Farrell had served as a school administrator in New York City. Edson (1906–1907), who was one of the superintendents in New York City, shared Farrell's view of special education. He emphasized that special education should be seen as a "productive expenditure" rather than "mere charity." Edson was impressed by the efficiency of the special education classrooms. He thought that this efficiency was validated by the fact that fewer children were being held back to repeat grades. Several years after Edson had made these observations, Fitts (1916) agreed with him that special education helped the entire school system. Looking back on the development of special education classes in Boston, Fitts recalled that these classes had been established "to relieve the [regular education] teacher who gives perhaps thirty per cent. [*sic*] of her energy to the few feeble-minded pupils she may have" (p. 78). Fitts urged the parents of children without disabilities to support special education. Otherwise, the attention that a regular teacher would devote to special learners would be "taken from her normal pupils."

Bicknell (1907), who was a professor at the University of Nebraska, agreed with those educators who detected system-wide benefits from special education.

Despite the force of these arguments, Bicknell feared that they would not be influential. He drew this conclusion after he had studied the national debate over special education. He believed that this debate was being dominated by partisans who were not concerned about the genuine interests of students. He characterized the partisans as "political adventurers" who wished to advance their personal interests or some ulterior cause. Although Bicknell believed that special education offered few opportunities for political meddling, he feared that this feature might turn out to be a disadvantage. Bicknell predicted that some elected politicians, once they realized that they only had limited chances to score partisan gains through special education, would refuse to fund it.

Writing during the same year as Bicknell, Rogers (1907) identified some the different educational resources that were available to persons with disabilities. He noted that these resources included professional educational associations. He explained that he was referring to "our association for the study of the feeble-minded, but also now our association for the study of backward and delinquent children" (p. 19). Physical facilities to house persons with disabilities constituted another important resource that was available to persons with disabilities. Some of the physical facilities were traditional, such as "institutions for the feeble-minded" and the "training schools for delinquent children" (p. 19). However, new types of facilities had begun to appear. These included group homes that were situated in communities and "special classes in the public schools" (p. 19). Although he wished to refrain from specifying the optimal type of facility, Rogers could not restrain himself. He suggested that "the state should provide permanent, village community homes" (p. 19).

Confrontational political actions often accompanied special education. Sometimes these actions were extremely complex. Dunlop (1912) was aware of complicated political dynamics when she wrote her exhaustive chronicle of child labor in Great Britain. Although she recognized that political factions had spurred educational progress, Dunlop also noted instances in which political factions had inhibited progress. She thought that three political groups had been particularly effective in delaying school reform. Industrialists, who worried about the rising expenses that they would incur if they relinquished their dependence on child labor, had opposed policies requiring universal school attendance. Parents who depended on the wages of children also had opposed progressive educational policies. Finally, fiscally conservative taxpayers, who realized that educational reforms required the construction of buildings, the hiring of teachers, and the expansion of operating budgets, opposed progressive policies.

Continuing Political Changes

During the decade prior to the 1920s, members of the public disagreed about whether the government should recognize the rights of disabled persons. Even those persons who favored some government-assured rights still argued among themselves about which rights should be recognized. They also argued about the services that the state should provide to persons with disabilities. Scholars participated in these arguments. Lapage (1911), who was a British physician, twisted his rhetoric in ways that revealed this confusion. While attempting to define the ideal system with which to manage and educate persons with disabilities, Lapage alternately pandered to extremists and reformers. He sided with the extremists when he stated that "efficient lifelong care and supervision" for persons with disabilities was "absolutely essential" (p. 238). Declaring that "the legal powers of controlling the feeble-minded are lamentably insufficient," he demanded that the government be authorized to register all disabled citizens. Lapage believed that this action was necessary so that the government could monitor disabled citizens effectively. Even though he substantively agreed with the extremists, Lapage did oppose them on several key issues. He strongly disagreed with those extremists who thought that special education lacked practical value. He also disagreed with those who insisted on universal, involuntary sterilization. Lapage wrote that involuntary sterilization was "neither desirable nor necessary, if efficient permanent care is enforced" (p. 238).

In Great Britain, citizens had been ambivalent about the appropriate way to treat disabled persons. The different factions of British educators had spent a great deal of energy feuding with each other. They also spent a great deal of energy in their efforts to persuade ambivalent citizens. Like their British counterparts, the American citizens were uncertain about the way to treat disabled persons. Like their British counterparts, American educators appealed to their ambivalent countrymen. For example, those educators who had confidence in special education attempted to attract allies. They even relied on the same rhetorical strategies that their British colleagues had employed. Claxton (1911), who was the United States Commissioner of Education, restated an argument that many British scholars had used. He warned his American audience that "school authorities have seen for many years that the presence of [children with disabilities] in the regular classes is detrimental to the progress of both the exceptional and the non-exceptional" (p. 5). Claxton contended that the expansion of special education would help students with disabilities and those without them.

Writing just a year after Claxton, Bolton (1912) was a special education advocate who attempted to engage critics through a somewhat oblique argument.

Realizing that some persons were disappointed with the results of special education, Bolton initially agreed with them. However, he cleverly pointed to the complex political factors that explained this failure. For example, he alleged that those teachers who worked within special institutions were "inferior in training and professional equipment to those engaged in our public schools" (p. 64). Bolton added several more comments, which were even more politically volatile.

> In many states a superintendent of a very small village might become a superintendent of a school for the blind or the deaf, if he knew how to pull political wires. Cast your eye over the country and see if the superintendents of the state schools for exceptional children as a class rank with the men of distinction in city superintendencies often paying smaller salaries? [*sic*] In the institutions for the feeble-minded the case is still worse. Barring the superintendent, the consulting physician, and the nurses, most of the attendants are of the servant class and in no way rank as real teachers. (p. 64)

To engender support for special educational programs, some advocates highlighted the accelerated rate at which these programs were being established. Wallin (1914), who was a professor at the University of Pittsburgh, informed his readers that the school leaders in approximately 350 cities already had established "special classes for the retarded, the seriously backward . . . and for the feeble-minded" (p. 13). However, Wallin (1915–1916) qualified the preceding remarks in one of his later publications. In that subsequent publication, he claimed that the misuse of standardized intelligence tests was one of the primary reasons that students were qualifying for special education. On the basis of this later analysis, Wallin concluded that many special education programs were not justified.

Kuhlmann (1915) was another scholar who highlighted the impressive rate at which special education programs had been proliferating. Like Wallin, Kuhlmann thought that ulterior factors had contributed to this growth. One of these factors was the "constant tendency to include higher and higher grade cases in the category of feeble-minded" (p. 215). Although he had observed the same phenomenon that Kuhlmann had, Campbell (1917a) interpreted it differently. In fact, Campbell was pleased that the range for disabilities had expanded. Campbell explained that this expansion provided the basis from which to reclassify many of the persons who had been labeled as delinquents and criminals but who truly were disabled.

Spaulding (1920), who was the Superintendent of the Cleveland schools, agreed with those contemporaries who acknowledged the rapidity with which special education programs were spreading. Furthermore, he did not conceal his reservations about that growth. He particularly worried that the money that had been diverted to special learners had not yielded enough results to justify that expenditure.

> How much can we afford to spend on the education of the feeble-minded?. . . . It is a fair question to ask whether we are doing as much good to all the people in the community by spending three or four or five times as much per child on these feeble-minded children, whose best advocates will admit that no very great achievement may be expected from them compared with the normal children. (p. 77)

Spaulding (1920) admitted that his writings on special learners had convinced some readers that he was a critic without a heart. He objected that this characterization had been unfair. He insisted that all of his opinions were defensible because they were based on 25 years of school administrative experience. He explained that, during his administrative tenure, he had been assured of "innumerable places where the expenditure . . . on these types of children might not be doubled and trebled to great and certain advantage" (p. 77). Although he conceded that he had opposed recommendations to spend more money on special education, Spaulding claimed that he never had questioned the value of special education itself. Rather, he had used skepticism as a tool with which to clarify special education's "relative value."

To the surprise of some observers, the shifting political attitudes that were evident during World War I benefited the special education movement. The difficulty they had analyzing the contemporary social dynamics may have contributed to their surprise. The wartime public had become convinced that the nation's security was connected to its industrial production. This awareness had persuaded it to expand the role of vocational preparation in the schools (Giordano, 2004). The acceptance of vocational education created a predisposition toward vocationally oriented special education. As a result, vocational preparation became a key attribute of special education.

After the war, physically and emotionally impaired veterans were referred to specialized rehabilitation programs. Some of these veterans resembled the children, adolescents, and adults in special education programs. As had been the case with vocational education, vocational rehabilitation predisposed the public toward special education. Davies (1923) characterized the wartime era and the years that followed it as the "modern period" of special education. He thought the period was characterized by "the development of an adequate program for dealing with the large numbers of mental defectives in the population" (p. 19). Davies added that this period also was marked by the adoption of multiple innovations, including "extra-institutional methods of care, training and supervision" (p. 19).

Individualized attention was an integral component of vocational education, vocational rehabilitation, and special education. Additionally, individualized attention was a concept that was becoming more popular among mainstream educators. Most of the mainstream educators who were drawn to individualized education demonstrated clearly defined humanistic propensities. Writing after the war, Woodrow (1919) asserted that this humanistic movement had been the primary source of special education. He wrote that special education was "part of the broader problem of adapting the school offerings as far as possible to the individual needs of all children, including the mediocre, [*sic*] or normal" (pp. 266–267). However, Woodrow tempered his desire to promote humanism with a desire to make precisely engineered social changes. Adopting a socialist philosophy, he recommended that each child "be trained to his maximal usefulness, and prepared to fit into his proper place in the social organization" (p. 310). Anticipating that his readers might be disconcerted by the way in which he had combined humanist and socialist ideologies, Woodrow attempted to explain his motive. He wrote that "social solidarity, the subordination of the individual to society, is not to be attained by attempting to make everyone alike" but instead "by adapting our educational methods in the case of each child to his capacity for serving society" (p. 310).

The national political mood toward persons with disabilities continued to evolve. As a result of the changes, some educators who had opposed special education reversed their stance. Walter Fernald, who was a Massachusetts school administrator, was an example. Fernald initially had cited eugenic evidence to justify the confinement of disabled persons in institutions. In one of his early reports, Fernald (1912) had applauded the "striking awakening of professional and popular consciousness of the widespread prevalence of feeble-mindedness . . . as a causative factor in the production of crime, prostitution, pauperism, illegitimacy, intemperance and other complex social diseases" (p. 87). Fernald thought that these endemic social problems resulted from a genetically transmitted "tendency." In fact, he assured his readers that "there is not doubt as to the potency and certainty of this hereditary tendency" (p. 88). On the basis of the preceding argument, Fernald adjured the public to disregard special education. Six years after he had made the preceding remarks, Fernald (1918) still maintained his early convictions. He chastised the public, which he thought was losing sight of the "eugenic" reasons for institutionalizing patients. Fernald lamented that the majority of patients were being committed "because they have become troublesome members of the community or because their care entails much difficulty under home conditions, with the eugenic considerations quite secondary" (p. 171).

Walter Fernald had been cynical about the value of educating persons with disabilities. However, Fernald (1923) underwent an ideological transformation. Taking advantage of the political momentum behind the programs to rehabilitate military veterans, Fernald became a spokesperson for special education. He attempted to win over recalcitrant colleagues through a complex argument. He began this rhetorical exercise with a series of observations. By extrapolating the army's intelligence testing data to the general population, Fernald calculated that 25,000,000 persons in the United States "were of decidedly inferior intelligence" (p. 399). He claimed that this estimate had been corroborated by educational authorities in his home state, Massachusetts. The Massachusetts authorities had recorded "the names and addresses of over 20,000 feeble-minded persons" (p. 399). Furthermore, they were "adding to that list at the rate of between 5,000 and 6,000 new names each year" (p. 399). On the basis of these data, Fernald concluded that disabled persons were not predestined to lives of social failure. Suspecting that his audience might have had difficulty extracting politically progressive lessons from his somewhat incoherent observations, he tried to assist them. Fernald explained that "there is something wrong in the old theory as to the probable fate of the defective person, because it is obvious that the majority of the subnormal children who have been considered in our school systems for the last two decades have been practically absorbed and assimilated by the community" (p. 399).

More and more of professional colleagues adopted the viewpoint that Fernald had represented. In fact, many of them were eager to demonstrate its validity. For example, Erickson (1931) cited data to discredit those American politicians who wished to establish a set of national eugenic standards. After examining 1500 convicts, Erickson concluded that the relationship between their aberrant behaviors and their "degree of feeble-mindedness was essentially without import" (p. 758).

Legal Issues

Concerned about the danger from persons with disabilities, many citizens supported legal and political actions to reduce that danger. In a report that they presented to a national conference on charities, Kerlin and Greene (1884) warned the delegates that a crisis was imminent. They explained that America's 1880 national census had revealed the presence of a "great army" of disabled persons. Kerlin and Greene worried because so few of the warriors from this army had been committed to institutions. In fact, they calculated that only three percent of disabled Americans had been institutionalized. Convinced that this situation was "not only detrimental to the individuals themselves, but subversive of the best interests of the family and neighborhood," Kerlin and Greene recommended universal institutionalization. They added that this plan was "not only a charitable, but [also] a conservative thing to do" (p. 15). Despite their belief in the need for extensive institutionalization, Kerlin and Greene recognized that the current asylums could not accommodate additional patients. They therefore recommended that government leaders build more asylums, "proceed to legislate for these defectives," and enforce universal institutionalization "on a permanent basis" (p. 15).

The citizens of Great Britain had anticipated the legal issues that the Americans were facing. In a lecture that he had delivered to Britain's Royal College of Physicians, Conolly (1850) had referred to the prevailing legal treatment of persons with disabilities. He believed that this treatment had been extremely unfair. After stating somewhat amorphously that "temporary excitement and social prejudices . . . render justice difficult," Conolly attempted to clarify this point. He hoped that a discussion of actual cases would be helpful. Most of his examples illustrated the different ways in which the social status or wealth of defendants had influenced the course of legal deliberations. Conolly noted that in any case involving a wealthy and upper-class defendant, "noble and distinguished persons [would] interfere to prevent his liberty being [*sic*] encroached upon" (p. 303). In contrast, persons from the lower social and economic classes routinely had been incarcerated. To redress this situation, Conolly encouraged barristers to voluntarily defend the many impoverished persons with disabilities who otherwise would be treated unjustly. Proclaiming that "the time for . . . revision must come," Conolly encouraged all of his readers to demand laws and court procedures that would protect the civil rights of all disabled persons.

Henderson (1901), who was a professor at the University of Chicago, acknowledged the degree to which Americans were indebted to their British colleagues. Writing originally in 1893, he discussed several ways that British advancements could improve the "social treatment" of Americans with disabilities. One of his central recommendations was that American citizens should model their legal practices after those that British citizens had been employing. Henderson explained that Americans should study England's "governing and guiding principles" for persons with disabilities and then extract "what is common to us with them" (p. iv).

In addition to admiring British laws, Henderson (1901) approved of those British educational programs that were government-funded and community-based. He employed rococo language to recapitulate the arguments that British advocates had used to advance these initiatives.

> The duty of caring for the poor of a community rests upon all, and its burden
> should be shared by all. This is impossible under the purely voluntary system,

where the avaricious escape and the liberal are doubly burdened. Under a system of taxation each citizen, except the dodgers of taxes, contributes according to his wealth and ability. The agents of the state, being clothed with legal authority, are in a better position to prevent imposition and deception than private citizens. It is said to be an advantage to include the charities of the people in one harmonious and complete system, in order to secure efficiency and economy. (pp. 58–60)

Henderson (1901) was aware that some persons did not admire the social theory to which British citizens had deferred. In fact, these critics alleged that Britain's social problems stemmed from the poorly conceived social foundation for British law. Henderson, who did not share the attitudes of the critics, applauded the general system of British law. He especially applauded those recent British statues that had affected disabled persons. Although he recognized that the British legal system had problems, Henderson reassured American readers that these problems were "based chiefly on defects in the law and its administration, defects which can be remedied without giving up the principle" (pp. 58–60).

Great Britain's Mental Deficiency Act

The European leaders who enacted legislation during the early part of the twentieth century wished to respond to their constituents. However, they had to be careful because those constituents were in the process of assuming new viewpoints toward disabled citizens. Great Britain's legislators were attentive to their most politically progressive constituents when they passed the *Mental Deficiency Act*. Writing during the year that the *Mental Deficiency Act* was passed, Wormald and Wormald (1913) described it as "the charter of a real liberty to a large number of chronic mentally defectives" (p. 91). In the preface to the book by Wormald and Wormald, Harvey (1913) noted that "hitherto, apart from the Elementary Education . . . Act, 1899, which . . . has not been adopted by many local authorities, the only method by which the community has offered assist [*sic*] . . . has been by voluntary charity or . . . the Poor Law" (p. vii).

Although its official purview did not extend beyond England's borders, the *Mental Deficiency Act* inspired advocates of persons with disabilities in other countries. The authors of the British law carefully had defined persons with disabilities, the ways in which they were to be treated, their rights to due process, and the governmental agencies that were responsible for them. After he had listed the educational and governmental organizations that were charged with meeting the needs of persons with disabilities, Young (1916) added that these units had been "called upon to assist in discovering" persons with disabilities. They also had been charged with "devising means for [disabled persons'] training, care and control" (p. v). Kirby (1914), who was the secretary of England's National Association for the Feeble-minded, commended this law for the rights that it defined and the sanctions that it established. She optimistically predicted that "after the passing of this Act no person will be disfranchised by reason of the maintenance of an institution, or under guardianship, [*sic*] of a defective for whom he is responsible" (p. 7).

Some political groups had opposed the *Mental Deficiency Act*. Harvey (1913) reported that this act elicited "strenuous opposition from a number of men and women" (p. ix). He explained that these opponents had been "eager to protect industrial liberty from from the growing power of officalism [*sic*]" (p. ix). This legal act also was opposed by those groups that wished to protect society from persons with disabilities. Sponsors of the law were aware of this resistance. They reassured the public that disabled persons would not be presented with a full set of legal safeguards. For example, Kirby (1914) explained that the *Mental Deficiency Act* provided only limited legal rights to disabled persons. In those cases in which British citizens were convicted of sexually abusing disabled individuals, the *Mental Deficiency Act* did authorize imprisonment. Nonetheless, judges could exclude "hard labor" from the offenders' sentences. In those cases in which citizens had abused females with disabilities, the law precluded the judges from imposing long sentences. Because of the widespread belief that females with disabilities invited sexual assaults, the judges only could detain offenders for periods that did not exceed two years.

Even though they were aware of the limitations of the *Mental Deficiency Act*, Wormald and Wormald (1913) judged that it was "a distinct step forward in the history of the treatment of mental deficiency" (p. 95). Young (1916), who was a British barrister, agreed with these scholars. To show his respect for the *Mental Deficiency Act*, Young included its entire text within his book. In spite of this respect, Young saw a need to apply the law cautiously. He thought that caution was necessary because of the many disputes in the field that were still unresolved. For example, the professionals in the health fields could not agree among themselves about the aptitudes and liabilities of persons with disabilities. To illustrate this point, Young pointed out that "there are several authorities who are agreed that . . . it is impossible to say before the age of 11 or 12 years (i.e. after 4 or 5 years' careful observation) whether a child will be able to earn its [*sic*] own living without control and supervision" (p. 98). Young did not conceal his own doubts about this issue. In fact, those doubts were revealed in the quotation that he selected for the conclusion of his book. The quotation was one from a British scholar who claimed that only one percent of special education students would be able to "earn their own livelihood in a separate existence in the outside world" (Dr. Caldecott, a physician assigned to the Earlswood Asylum, n.d., as quoted by Young, 1916, p. 98).

Laws Affecting the Civil Rights of Americans With Disabilities

Like the citizens of Great Britain, the residents of the United States began to view persons with disabilities differently. Their changing views created legal and educational problems. Cornell and Ross (1928) underscored this point in their historical analysis of American special education. They identified the period from 1910–1920 as one in which many laws affecting persons with disabilities had been enacted. However, Cornell and Ross judged that the lawmakers of this era had generated political friction through some of the legal enactments. One of the reasons the lawmakers created friction was their failure to fully appreciate the public's new mood toward persons with disabilities. Cornell and Ross emphasized that "the public attitude toward the problem of mental deficiency" was undergoing "considerable change" (p. 82). Cornell and Ross added that the once-prevalent "alarmist" attitudes were being replaced by more moderate convictions.

Schlapp (1915) had anticipated the comments that Cornell and Ross (1928) would articulate more than a decade later. Schlapp had been worried about the professionals who managed the criminal justice system. He feared that they lacked the training to deal with a society that had become politically more progressive. Schlapp specifically was concerned that many judges, police officers, and truant officers would be unable to evaluate the degrees to which disabilities had influenced the behaviors of the delinquents with whom they interacted. Although he was distressed by the problems in the criminal justice system, Schlapp was ever more worried about those in the educational system, where the pace of change was slower still. Because of this inertia, Schlapp adjured his readers to promote social and political changes on all fronts. He explained that rapid progress was necessary "for anything approaching justice . . . to be done, or anything approaching efficiency and protection of society . . . to be achieved" (p. 185).

Like Schlapp, Doll (1917) recognized that the judges and other law-enforcement authorities were facing significant challenges. Unlike Schlapp, Doll believed that these authorities could handle the challenges. He wrote that the authorities had been "rapidly adjusting legal and personal responsibility to individual mental capacity" (p. 5). Doll added that the law-enforcement authorities had abandoned "the notion that political equality signifies intellectual equality in our democratic society" (p. 5). By discarding antiquated political ideology, they had prepared themselves for a philosophy of education that "demands that instruction and the course of study be adjusted to the pupil's individual learning capacity" (p. 6). Doll concluded that the actions of the law-enforcement authorities were being copied by other groups, including "our leading psychologists, educators, sociologists and eugenists [*sic*]" (p. 6).

Kuhlmann (1915), Anderson (1915–1916), and many other scholars had alluded to the legal complications that had resulted from society's shifting attitudes toward persons with disabilities. Some of these legal problems were the consequence of the extremely specific fashion in which some state lawmakers had constrained persons with disabilities. Wallin (1922a) made this point about Missouri's lawmakers.

> Among the laws that have been enacted [between 1915 and 1922 by Missouri lawmakers] are the following: the imposition of a penalty on the county clerks for failure to report deaf and blind children to the state institutions for the deaf and blind . . .; extending the compulsory years of age to the proper state institutions; extending the compulsory attendance law to feeble-minded, blind, deaf and crippled children; authorization of the establishment of special public school classes . . .; and prohibiting the marriage of the imbecile, feeble-minded, insane and epileptic, and providing a fine of not less than $500 or imprisonment in a county jail not exceeding one year, or both, for solemnizing such a marriage. (Wallin, 1922a, p. 121)

The distinctive laws that were passed in each state may not have accurately depicted the philosophies, values, and attitudes of the citizens in those states. However, those laws did reveal the distinctive philosophies, values, and attitudes of their legislators. Hamilton and Haber (1917) wrote a book in which they attempted to recapitulate the ways in which persons with disabilities had been affected by diverse state laws. In the introduction to that monograph, Haber (1917) admitted that "with the exception of the laws of a few of the leading states . . . the laws presented a chaotic mass, which it has been exceedingly difficult to survey" (p. vii). Haber added that "in many instances the laws of certain states contain enactments of which counterparts are not found in others" (p. viii).

Idiosyncratic state laws sometime challenged and at other times advanced the interests of disabled citizens. To underscore this unevenness, Hamilton and Haber (1917) analyzed each state law affecting persons with disabilities. To simplify their state-by-state analysis, they used a common set of topical headings, such as those laws that pertained to special education, sterilization, and marriage. The manner in which they proceeded was exemplified in their summary of the marriage laws in Kansas.

No woman under the age of forty-five years or man of any age, except he marry a woman over forty-five years, either of whom is epileptic, imbecile, or feeble-minded, may marry any persons within the state. (Hamilton & Haber, 1917, p. 70)

Hamilton and Haber (1917) contrasted the marriage laws of Kansas with those of New Jersey.

Feebleminded and epileptic persons who have been confined in any public institution for their care or treatment may not marry without obtaining a certificate from two licensed physicians, that they are entirely cured and that there is little probability that the defects will be transmitted to the issue of the marriage. (Hamilton & Haber, 1917, pp. 142–143)

As for the marriage laws of Louisiana, Hamilton and Haber declared simply that "the statutes make no mention of the feebleminded or of the epileptic" (p. 76).

Anderson and Fearing (1923) believed that positive and negative assumptions had a great impact on the ways in which persons with disabilities were treated. Furthermore, they believed that many of these negative assumptions were unfounded. They thought that legislators had compounded this situation by using unfounded, negative assumptions as the basis for their laws. Although they thought that the legislators had deferred to numerous groups, Anderson and Fearing accused them of being especially deferential to poorly trained researchers. They claimed that these incompetent researchers had employed biased samples within their studies. Anderson and Fearing concluded that "most of the legislation in this field has been based on generalizations from studies of striking failures, such as feebleminded criminals, feeble-minded vagrants, feebleminded prostitutes, and feebleminded dependents" (p. 3).

During the first two decades of the twentieth century, scholars detected shifting political attitudes towards disabled persons. East (1923) identified one of the multiple legal complications that these shifts had produced. After noting that more and more instances of mental illness were being linked to disabilities, East warned that this trend would have an impact on criminal prosecutions. He was especially concerned about cases in which "insanity and mental deficiency are combined in a person accused of a serious crime" (p. 157). East had specific advice for the scholars, psychologists, and medical personnel who would appear as expert witnesses in court cases. He anticipated that they would be asked to differentiate the aspects of a defendant's behavior that were associated with mental deficiency from those aspects that were attributable to mental illness. East warned professionals that they would create "awkward" impressions if they were not prepared to resolve this problem when they confronted it in courtrooms.

In a report that they published during the 1920s, Town and Hill (n.d.) gave specific examples of politically progressive initiatives that had been benefiting persons with disabilities. For example, they presented information about alternative living facilities for disabled persons. Town and Hill identified states in which the political climate had facilitated the development of alternative facilities. They also identified states in which the political climate had restricted the emergence of alternative facilities. They singled out Massachusetts as a state in which the political climate had been particularly advantageous for persons with disabilities. Town and Hill explained that "in 1921 a law was passed providing for the commitment of feebleminded persons to the custody of the Department of Mental Disease, which department has the option of placing the committed person in an institution or of supervising him in the community" (p. 283). Town and Hill added that the new Massachusetts practices were "in the spirit of the British practice" (p. 283).

Town and Hill (n.d.) did not conceal their personal support for community-based facilities, which they judged to be more effective than prisons or asylums. To underscore the rationale for that support, they presented a set of diagrams. These diagrams represented the high rate of recidivism among the disabled criminals who had been released from restrictive facilities. Figure 5.1, which contains one of these diagrams, was intended to help readers see the benefits of community-based facilities. However, this diagram was so complicated that it may have confused rather than helped readers.

Writing about the same time as Town and Hill (n.d.), Walter Fernald (1923) was struck by the Massachusetts legislation that protected the disabled citizens in that state. Fernald highlighted a 1921 Massachusetts law "requiring that every school child three, four or more years retarded shall be given a mental examination, and also providing that such children must be given special training" (p. 399). Fernald was aware that the public's shifting attitudes had provided the supporters of this law with substantial political leverage. He wrote that the attitudes of earlier generations had been based upon "generalizations and deductions concerning the feeble-minded" that were "far too sweeping" (p. 398). In contrast, Fernald thought that the emerging views were based on the careful "study of the mentally defective in special school classes, school clinics, outpatient mental clinics, in private practice, in community surveys and in the army tests" (p. 398).

The citizens of Massachusetts had demonstrated changed political attitudes toward special education. Fernald (1923) applauded the state leaders of Massachusetts for the exemplary manner in which they had responded to these changed attitudes. Even though they initially may have developed programs in response to pressure from their constituents, the state leaders eventually used the success of those

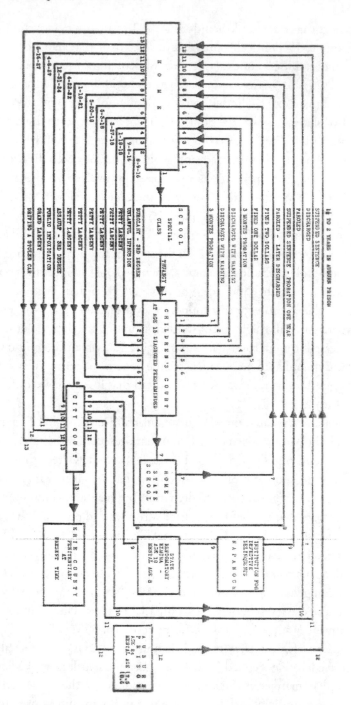

Figure 5.1. Early Twentieth-Century Diagram Intended to Highlight the Benefits of Community-Based Facilities.

programs to engender broader support for special education. To substantiate this point, Fernald informally assessed the extent to which the citizens of Massachusetts were receptive of special education. His observations convinced him that Massachusetts citizens demonstrated extraordinary sensitivity to special learners. Fernald noted that "to-day in Massachusetts little attention is paid to the defective until he behaves badly or gets into trouble" (p. 399). Fernald concluded that "the majority of the subnormal children [in Massachusetts] who have been considered in our school systems for the last two decades have been practically absorbed and assimilated by the community" (p. 399).

Legislation Affecting Public Special Education

Prior to the 1920s, few state leaders paid attention to special education. When Hamilton and Haber (1917) searched for instances of state-regulated special education systems, they could locate only seven examples. Some of these cases involved laws that were relatively detailed. For example, Oklahoma's laws delineated a curriculum of sorts. The Oklahoma legislators had instructed the special educators in their state to emphasize the "agriculture and mechanical arts, the English language and the various branches of mathematical, physical, and economical science, with special reference to application in the industries of life" (Hamilton & Haber, 1917, p. 174). The lawmakers in several states had identified the government office that was responsible for the education of children with disabilities. Although the lawmakers in Michigan and Oregon did not identify a state office, they did describe the manner in which disabled children were to be reported to local educational authorities.

From state to state, the laws that affected special education exhibited varying degrees of precision. Consider the detailed language in a politically progressive statute that was enacted by Connecticut legislators in 1919.

> No educationally exceptional child may be disbarred from school attendance except on the approval of the Director of the Division of Special Education and Standards and of the Commissioner of Education; and every child whose exclusion is thus approved shall immediately be brought to the attention of the Bureau of Child Welfare, and said Bureau shall report the case with recommendations to the selectmen of the town in which the child is legally resident; and shall take any further action necessary to insure adequate protection and training for the child. (Passage from a Connecticut law, 1919, as quoted by Gesell, 1921, p. 62)

The preceding statute was not the only politically progressive law that state legislators enacted during this period. In 1919, Pennsylvania's legislators adopted a law to ensure that the children with disabilities in their state would have access to special education. They even provided part of the funding for their education.

> An amendment to the school code was passed which requires that "each child— between the ages of eight and sixteen years—who is gravely retarded in his or her school work, or who, because of apparent exceptional physical or mental condition, is not being properly educated and trained," shall be examined and a report made to the proper authorities . . . that special classes in the public schools or special public schools shall be maintained for those who are fit subjects; and that the state shall pay half the expense. (Passage from a Pennsylvania law, 1919, as quoted and paraphrased by Abbot, 1920, p. 320)

The enactment of regulatory laws did not ensure that the lives of children and adults with disabilities would improve. It did not even ensure that those lives would change. Abbott and Breckinridge (1917) made this point after state lawmakers enacted a law requiring that children in Illinois attend school. To determine that law's impact, Abbott and Breckinridge studied the pattern of school attendance by students in Chicago and its neighboring vicinities. Before revealing the results of their research, they observed that "thirty-three years have passed since the principle of compulsory school attendance was adopted in the state of Illinois" (p. vii). Despite the significant length of this period, Abbott and Breckinridge presented extensive data to demonstrate "how slow we were to adopt this principle and how reluctantly, after it was adopted, the local educational authorities of the various towns, and counties to whom its enforcement was intrusted [*sic*], proceeded to act under it" (pp. vii–viii).

Several factors explained why local school administrators did not implement the state laws that regulated special education. Sometimes the school administrators had views that were different from those of their legislators. Even when they personally agreed with their legislators, they may have been restrained by unsympathetic constituencies. Sometimes they delayed implementation because they could not alter the considerable inertia of the educational bureaucracy. Sometimes they delayed because they did not have the classroom teachers that they needed to make changes. Sometimes limited budgets forced administrators to delay implementation. Because most of the laws regulating special education did not penalize districts that failed to comply, school administrators could delay implementation indefinitely.

The inadequacy of educational budgets was a perennial problem. Few state leaders had made the financing of special education a priority. Connecticut's lawmakers, who had agreed to pay half of the cost of special education programs, had set a positive example. Legislators in New Jersey also provided a positive example. Hamilton and Haber (1917) discussed some of the financial provisions of the New Jersey special education law.

> A sum, not exceeding $300 for each person, is appropriated each year for the education of such feebleminded persons as may be designated by the governor. If the parents are not able to pay the expense of clothing the pupil, an additional sum not exceeding thirty dollars per annum may be granted. If the person is sent out of the state, a sum not exceeding $400, including clothing, may be allowed. If sent to a hospital, $450 may be allowed. (p. 141).

Some of the state laws that mandated special services and special education failed to change the lives of persons with disabilities. These failures resulted from general factors such as social resistance and bureaucratic inertia. They also resulted from practical circumstances such as inadequate budgets and a shortage of trained personnel. Reformers blamed the bureaucrats in state agencies and the administrators in local school districts for not addressing these problems. Eliot (1925) believed that sometimes this blame had been inappropriate. He attributed a portion of the failures to those parents or guardians who were uninformed about educational opportunities. He attributed another portion of the failures to those parents or guardians who ignored the educational opportunities that were available to their children.

Eliot (1925) thought that additional state laws were needed to address the educational problems associated with parental neglect. He recommended laws that would empower educational administrators to take action without the support of the parents or caregivers. For example, he urged that school administrators be authorized to gain court assistance "in carrying out treatment or securing a change of treatment" for students with disabilities. The type of legislation that Eliot was recommending would have been extraordinarily intrusive. Eliot was aware that many citizens would be disquieted by this feature of his proposal. Therefore, Eliot reassured his readers that the "the majority of children being treated by special services of the educational system would . . . be on a voluntary basis" and that only "a few would be under treatment by court order" (p. 67).

Several years after Eliot (1925) had made his suggestions, Wallin (1933) commented on the enduring underutilization of special education. Wallin referred to a national conference of special educators at which the delegates had agreed on this precise point. On the basis of their observations and experiences, the conference participants had concluded that "over 90% of handicapped children in the schools of the United States who should be placed in special classes or be provided with special educational treatment are still retained in the regular grades" (p. 145).

In spite of the increasing opportunities that were available to them, the disabled children in many communities lacked access to special education programs. During the 1920s, some of these children attended regular education classrooms. However, even the opportunity to participate in regular education was uncertain. After he had examined recent court decisions, Edwards (1933) concluded that "no pupil has the right to attend [regular education classes] if his presence in the school impairs its efficiency or interferes with the rights of other pupils" (p. 506). Edwards gave the example of a Wisconsin child who had been transferred from a regular education classroom to one for children with communication problems. The student in question did not have difficulty hearing, speaking, or using language. Instead, he "had an uncontrolled flow of saliva, which drooled from his mouth on to his clothing and books, causing him to present an unclean appearance" (p. 507). The parents objected to the new scholastic placement because their child "seemed to be normal mentally" and to exhibit "fair progress in his studies" (p. 507). They explained that the highly specialized instruction in the new classroom was less appropriate than that which their son had been receiving in the regular education classroom. Because the problem could not be resolved amicably, the parents initiated a legal action against the school administrators. Eventually, this case was decided by the Supreme Court of Wisconsin, which supported the actions that the school administrators had taken. Edwards wrote that the judges had sanctioned the student's exclusion from regular education because the child "produced a depressing and nauseating effect upon both teacher and pupils . . . took up an undue portion of the teacher's time and attention, distracted the attention of other pupils, and interfered generally with the discipline and progress of the school" (p. 507).

Edwards (1933) described another case in which the administrators in a Massachusetts school district had barred a disabled student from regular education. They had judged that the child had been disruptive, uncouth, and insufficiently responsive to instruction. The parents were upset about the way in which these school administrators had treated their child. They also were upset about some of the allegations that the administrators had made about their child. They requested that a jury decide whether the allegations had merit. The Massachusetts Supreme Court, which eventually reviewed this case, confirmed the appropriateness of the school administrators' actions. Furthermore, it refused to honor the parent's request to allow a jury to validate the administrators' allegations.

> Whether certain acts of disorder so seriously interfere with the school that one who persists in them, either voluntarily or by reason of imbecility, should not be permitted to continue in the school, is a question which the statute makes it [the school administrators'] duty to answer, and if they answer honestly in an effort

to do their duty, a jury composed of men of no special fitness to decide educational questions should not be permitted to say that their answer is wrong. (Passage from *Watson v. City of Cambridge*, 157, Mass. 561, 32 N. E. 864, as quoted by Edwards, 1933, p. 508)

Edwards (1933) anticipated that his readers would compare the scholastic treatment of children with disabilities with the treatment of children from racial minority groups. However, Edwards detected a fundamental difference between these two situations. He stated emphatically that it had been "well established by many cases decided by both state and federal courts that legislation providing for separate schools for white and colored children does not violate any of the provisions of the federal constitution" (p. 508). Eventually, the courts would change their views about the educational rights of students from racial minority groups. They also would shift the way in which they had been viewing students with disabilities.

The school administrators who attempted to implement special education were restricted by complicated social and political situations. They also were impeded by inadequate funding. Keesecker (1933) commented on the relationship between educational innovations and funding. He observed that "since the beginning of statehood in practically all of our States [*sic*] both legal and educational doctrines have regarded education as a State [*sic*] function" (p. 67). He immediately added that "State [*sic*] responsibility has been confined mostly to matters of administration rather than financial support of education" (p. 67). Keesecker judged that in 1922 this dysfunctional situation began to change. He wrote that 1922 was the year in which Delaware became "the first State to assume major responsibility for the support of public education" (p. 67). Zook (1934), who served later as the United States Commissioner of Education, designated several recent political changes that had affected schooling. He thought that one of these changes had been truly momentous. Zook had been referring to the increasing willingness of state legislators to pair demands for educational progress with funding.

Writing toward the end of the twentieth century, Sales, Powell, and Duziend (1982) took an historical look at the social and legal status of citizens from minority groups. Although they judged that this status had changed substantially for those persons who came from racial minority groups, these scholars concluded that disabled persons had "largely been left out of efforts in recent years to guarantee the rights of minority groups" (p. 9). Commenting specifically on several court cases, Sales, Powell, and Duziend noted that only recently had some of the enduring legal problems of disabled citizens been addressed. The three researchers presented an example of one judge who had drawn a conclusion about any disabled person who was depicted as a threat to the community. This judge had affirmed the right of the accused person "to challenge the allegation before a neutral decisionmaker [*sic*] prior to deprivation of his or her rights" (p. 9). Sales, Powell, and Duziend applauded this judge for confirming that "basic, fundamental rights are essential for all persons" (p. 9). In spite of the progress that they detected, the three scholars judged that the rights of many persons with disabilities still were compromised. They predicted that future political campaigns would attempt to redress this situation.

Summary

Throughout the nineteenth and twentieth centuries, politically diverse groups argued about the amount of liberty that was appropriate for persons with disabilities. The disputants included scholars, physicians, lawmakers, educators, and members of the general public. These groups also debated about special education. Some of them thought that special education was an idealistic venture that would not be effective. Others thought that it was too expensive or too dangerous. The supporters rejoined that special education increased the quality of participants' lives, lowered the need for costly social services, reduced crime, and promoted independence. They shored up their claims with examples of disabled children and adults who had been helped through education. Attracted by the mixture of humanitarian and economic arguments, more and more persons endorsed special education. They acknowledged the need for laws to define, codify, and disseminate it.

Epilogue: A Revolutionary Law

[Each state must have] a policy that assures all handicapped children the right to a free appropriate public education.
                    —Education for All Handicapped Children Act, 1975

Many groups joined the 1970s campaign to help persons with disabilities. The participants included parents, caregivers, community leaders, teachers, physicians, scientists, lawyers, judges, lawmakers, businesspersons, journalists, and social activists. Although their larger goal was to help all disabled persons, they focused their efforts on students in the schools. They supported fresh definitions of disabilities, innovative assessment techniques, and novel types of remediation. They lobbied for legislation to disseminate and secure these scholastic changes.

Continued Dissatisfaction With Special Education

During the early part of the twentieth century, educational reformers repeatedly had called attention to the problems that disabled learners faced. At mid century, they had not relented. At a 1952 conference on special education, two federal officials (Reed & Jones, 1957) characterized these problems as pervasive and profound. Furthermore, they predicted that the problems would endure. One of the reasons that the officials were so pessimistic was the bickering in which educators engaged. They pointed out that this feuding had impeded the establishment of a coherent political agenda. Although some of the matters over which the educators had wrangled were petty, others were substantive. As an example of a somewhat substantive procedural issue, the officials noted that the educators had been unable to decide "whether the provision of school services for [children with disabilities] is a function of the public schools or of public welfare agencies" (Reed & Jones, 1957, p iii).

Hill (1957), who was a federal educational authority, had participated in the 1952 conference at which two of his colleagues had made their forecast about the dismal fate awaiting special education. Not as gloomy as his colleagues, Hill applauded some of the achievements of special educators. For example, he noted that they currently were educating more children with disabilities than ever before. Even though he did detect progress, Hill also detected genuine problems. He speculated that all special education students, even if one included those who were registered in private schools, would comprise only 15 percent of the children who were eligible for these programs. Anticipating that some of his readers might question this allegation, Hill added defensively that "no one knows how many [children with disabilities] are not in any school at all" (p. 1). As for the reason that most disabled children were not enrolled in special classes, Hill conjectured that qualified instructors and suitable facilities were not available.

Hill (1957) had been concerned about the number of children with disabilities who were not enrolled in special education programs. He had made his remarks at a federal conference that had been convened in the 1950s. During this era, Samuel Kirk and two associates (Kirk, Karnes, & Kirk, 1955) had developed a manual in which they advised parents about the educational opportunities that were available to children with disabilities. In the second edition of that manual, which they published 13 years after the initial publication, the authors (Kirk, Karnes, & Kirk, 1968) noted that "enrollment in institutional and public school programs had increased tremendously" since 1955. Although they were impressed by this growth, the authors concluded that special education was undersubscribed. They estimated that only 400,000 mentally retarded children had been instructed in the public schools during 1967.

Gardner and Warren (1978) were scholars who examined students' access to special education during the 1960s. Like many other scholars, they concluded that a significant number of children with disabilities had been denied suitable educational opportunities during this period. Gardner and Warren judged that this problem that had been festering for a long time. Nonetheless, they did discern efforts to expand access to special education during the 1960s. In spite of these efforts, the problem had not been resolved. They opined that "by 1970, only about one half of the number of children estimated to need special education in the United States were [*sic*] receiving it" (p. 42). Gardner and Warren then added a cautionary qualification. They pointed out that they had used national statistics from the 1960s to estimate whether children had access to special education. These data had revealed a "marked variation in different state systems of education in the degree to which exceptional children received service" (p. 42). As a result of these early variations in state practices, some exceptional learners had been assigned to classes that were far from appropriate. Gardner and Warren judged that inappropriate assignments had been made so often and so extensively that the resulting damage could not be eliminated for some time.

Gardner and Warren (1978) had referred to regional influences on the ways that special learners were treated. Prior to the enactment of the *Education for All Handicapped Children Act*, the lawmakers and bureaucrats from different states had employed extremely variable definitions of disabilities. As a result, the laws and regulations that they had created often confused their constituencies. Educators, parents, and members of the public, who could not appeal to a national standard when they were grouping and identifying students, argued among themselves about which students should qualify for special education. They were especially contentious when they were deliberating about students with mild disabilities. Although mild educational disability was a relatively new diagnostic category in the schools, it was being assigned more frequently than any other category of disability. Critics demanded that learners with mild disabilities be treated in a consistent and professional manner.

Like many other educators, Kolstoe (1972) was disconcerted by the controversies surrounding mildly handicapped learners. He reported that "there have appeared in the literature numerous writings from diverse sources which suggest that provisions for children who show mild mental retardation do more harm than good" (p. 51). Kolstoe paraphrased some of the salient criticisms that had been made about the identification and treatment of learners with mild disabilities. For example, the critics had alleged that these learners, who had been diagnosed spuriously and branded with stereotypical labels, had been sent to programs in which they were separated from their peers and instructed inappropriately. Disoriented by inappropriate placements and instruction, the learners had set low academic expectations for themselves. Even though Kolstoe advised his readers that these problems were substantive, he assured them that they could be solved. He explained that "the present criticisms aimed at special classes are not so much criticism of the classes as they are criticisms of some of the administrative aspects of the program" (p. 51). To solve the problems to which he had referred, Kolstoe recommended changes in the ways that children with mild disabilities were identified and instructed.

During the 1960s and 1970s, many critics were displeased with the prevailing practices in special education. Some of them charged that flawed identification procedures had caused erroneous diagnoses of children from racial minority groups. When the misdiagnosed students were then restricted to special programs, the result was *de facto* segregation. Hoffman (1975) acknowledged that this criticism had influenced the course of legal proceedings. He reported that "it has been argued . . . with increasing success before the courts, that children of non-white, lower economic backgrounds are being misplaced into stigmatory [*sic*] and educationally inferior tracks for the mentally retarded or emotionally disturbed/socially maladjusted" (pp. 415–416).

Wishing to challenge the critics of special education, Hoffman (1975) reviewed some of the current laws and regulations affecting special learners. He concluded that every state had "enacted legislation, either mandatory or permissive, providing for the establishment of local school services for [children with disabilities]" (p. 416). Hoffman added that a comprehensive system of special education already had evolved. He detected not only services but also the funding that was required to sustain and further develop those services. Although Hoffman believed that progress had transpired, he did admit that many critics disagreed with him. These critics discerned differences between the educational services that were mandated and those that simply were encouraged. The critics were even angry about some of the mandated special education services because they thought these had been funded inadequately.

Like other scholars during the mid 1970s, Kirp, Buss, and Kuriloff (1974) attempted to assess the influence of current politics on education. They observed that many parents of children with disabilities were frustrated by the slow pace at which the educational bureaucracy had been addressing inappropriate educational practices. As a last resort, these parents had initiated legal actions. Kirp, Buss, and Kuriloff concluded that lawyers had "assumed an increasingly active role in disputes over the adequacy of education for the handicapped, promoting particular policy goals both through legislation and in test case litigation" (p. 40).

After they had documented some of the problems in the current system of special education, Kirp, Buss, and Kuriloff (1974) expressed their support for the citizens who were frustrated by those problems. They even supported those persons who had initiated legal actions to redress their problems. They also supported those critics who had called for legislation to redress the problems. Kirp, Buss, and Kuriloff endorsed a wide range of legislative acts. They encouraged legislation that would define disabled learners' rights to due process. They also wanted laws requiring parents to sign documents about the types of instruction that their children would receive. They endorsed laws authorizing alternative educational treatments.

They recommended laws empowering parents to bill school districts for educational services from other school districts or private companies. They encouraged federal lawmakers to set high educational standards, link those standards to legislation, and then provide the funding to implement that legislation.

A Law of Epic Proportions

The authors of Public Law 94–142 had asserted that "the special educational needs of handicapped children are not being fully met" (Education for All Handicapped Children Act, 1975, p. 1). Although they did not reveal the basis for this allegation, they claimed that "one million of the handicapped children in the United States are excluded entirely from the public school system" (p. 1). Congress passed Public Law 94–142 in 1975; President Ford signed it shortly thereafter.

The sponsors of Public Law 94–142 had highlighted some of the difficulties that disabled learners confronted. They also suggested ways to immediately reduce and eventually eliminate those difficulties. Although they believed that the education of children with disabilities should remain primarily the responsibility of the states, they encouraged the federal government to provide greater assistance to the states. Funding was one clear way to provide this assistance. In fact, many states needed financial help before they could improve or expand any of their special educational services.

The crafters of Public Law 94–142 did not think the federal government should limit its assistance to funding. They required it to create a national template for special education. This template would define the educational rights of persons with disabilities and the services to which they were entitled. It would assure that all public school districts were providing free and appropriate special education. It would guarantee that state and local educators were respecting due process, developing individualized educational programs, and employing uniform procedures. With regard to uniform procedures, the national template would specify the acceptable ways to identify, evaluate, and instruct children with disabilities.

The *Education for All Handicapped Children Act* was enacted in 1975. It was not implemented until 1977. At the time that it was signed, the sponsors had recognized that the states needed funds to implement it. Nonetheless, they had a hard time finding those funds. One of the reasons for this difficulty was the high priority that they had assigned to other educational projects. Cronin (1976) identified some of the popular educational projects that competed with the *Education for All Handicapped Children Act*. These priorities included the extension of vocational training and sex equality training. They also included the elimination of educational segregation, expansion of instructional television, support for the fine arts, acceleration of teacher preparation, and increased reliance on program assessment. After acknowledging that federal spending amounted to only 10 percent of the nation's total educational budget in the middle 1970s, Cronin noted that this contribution was enormously important to many states.

The *Education for All Handicapped Children Act* required every state to offer comprehensive services to students with disabilities. Braddock (1987) agreed with those analysts who judged that the cost of implementing this law had been compounded by the cost of implementing other federal educational initiatives. Furthermore, many persons viewed the expenses of Public Law 94–142 in the context of recent federal laws which, even though they were not focused on education, still had advanced the interests of persons with disabilities. Like the recent educational laws, those other laws had been funded inadequately. Congressional members, who apparently discerned these intertwining budgetary commitments, did provide a portion of the money for previously enacted and current mandates. As a result, the annual expenditures for the education and the healthcare of persons with disabilities increased dramatically. In fact, this category of federal funding grew by 200 percent from 1975–1980. Braddock (1987) thought that this budgetary trend would have continued if Ronald Reagan had not been elected president. Braddock concluded that this politically conservative president decisively changed the pattern of federal spending.

Increased funding was one characteristic of the *Education for All Handicapped Children Act*. An expanded regulatory scope was another characteristic. Even though legislators extended the scope of the new federal law beyond that of antecedent legislation, earlier legislators had anticipated some of the law's fiscal and regulatory features. Braddock (1987) elaborated on this point.

> Governmental programs are rooted in the past. Federal programs are rarely created totally anew, but rather are usually grafted to existing statutory and administrative structures. To understand current federal policy in mental retardation/developmental disabilities . . . one must be familiar with the historical record of myriad individual federal . . . program elements, and one must also appreciate each individual element's relation to its broader programmatic environment, its fiscal context, and its legislative history. (p. 1)

In the preceding passage, Braddock (1987) had referred to the historical pattern that had characterized the enactment of legislation. Aware that this pattern was changing, Braddock and other scholars contrasted the astonishing progress of the 1970s with the limited progress of other eras. Even though PL 94–142 was a federal initiative, it reflected practices that some states already had implemented. To demonstrate this point, Sarason and Doris (1979) compared the basic concepts in the 1975 *Education for All Handicapped Children Act* with those in Chapter 766, which was a 1972 Massachusetts law. Sarason and Doris referred to a *New York Times* reporter who had summarized features of the Massachusetts law.

> Chapter 766 discourages the labeling of handicapped children as much because of the "stigmatizing effect" this can have and instead emphasizes the individual needs of each child, determined through a "core evaluation" by a team consisting of a psychologist or social worker, doctor, or nurse, the child's present or most recent teacher, and a parent. The law mandates the involvement of parents and lay group in "overseeing, evaluating, and operating special education programs." (D. Milofsky, 1977, as quoted by Sarason & Doris, 1979, p. 376)

Although the citizens of Massachusetts had anticipated provisions of the *Education for All Handicapped Children Act*, the residents of many other states saw it as a revolutionary law. Sarason and Doris (1979) wrote that the changes that the federal law initiated were "of such variety and force, of such potential significance . . . [and] such speed, that one is hard put to account for them" (p. ix). Most persons who observed the effects of this law were as amazed as these two authors.

Many persons regarded the *Education for All Handicapped Children Act* as a landmark piece of legislation. How did the sponsors of this law gather the support that they needed to pass it? Attempting to answer this question, some scholars searched for clues in the radical political atmosphere of the 1970s. Writing during the 1970s, Hoffman (1975) linked recent educational changes to a long series of social developments. However, he also linked them to the distinctive style of advocacy that the parents of disabled children had been displaying lately. Hoffman believed that the extensive and intense efforts of parents decisively had influenced the course of special education.

In addition to studying the political atmosphere of the 1970s, some scholars examined that of the preceding decade. Sigmon (1987) was a scholar who thought that the 1960s might contain an explanation of the *Education for All Handicapped Children*. Although he had linked the enactment of the 1975 law to events from multiple decades, Sigmon concluded that the 1960s had been an extraordinarily important era. He pointed out that the contemporaries of this period had challenged the effectiveness of the prevalent special educational practices. They then had searched for alternatives to those practices. The *Education for All Handicapped Children Act* was the law that defined, funded, regulated, and promulgated those alternatives.

Like many of their professional colleagues, Sage and Burello (1986) were amazed at the educational changes of the 1970s. Like their colleagues, they wondered how such profound changes could have transpired in a short period. Sage and Burello concluded that numerous interrelated events had been responsible. They explained that "the decade of the 1970s brought to the field dynamic change, as reflected in public attitudes, enabling legal actions and everyday practices in the service system" (p. xiii). Winzer (1993) later agreed with the conclusion at which Sage and Burello had arrived. Even though he conceded that progress of the 1970s was connected to a complex series of antecedent events, Winzer insisted that events of the 1970s had been remarkable catalysts. Like other scholars, Winzer was particularly impressed by the intense and unrelenting lobbying of parents during the 1970s.

Although parents were unquestionably effective, they were aided by the other groups that joined them. For example, educators and journalists supported them. These groups generated great publicity when they testified about the cruel ways in which disabled children and adults were treated (e.g. Blatt & Kaplan, 1966; Blatt, 1973; Rivera, 1972). Blatt, who was a prominent special educator, was aware that the public's attitudes were malleable. In the foreword to a collection of essays that he had written during the 1960s and 1970s, he noted that "if there has been a revolution in the field of mental retardation over the past two or three decades, it has been not in the solution of its fundamental problems but in their perception" (Blatt, 1981, p. vii). To clarify this point, Blatt noted that more and more members of the public were viewing the "segregation, dehumanization, and even physical abuse" of persons with disabilities as the direct result of the prevailing "technology of treatment." Agreeing wholeheartedly with these sentiments, Blatt declared that restrictive hospitals, asylums, and treatment centers "inevitably produce dehumanization and abuse in spite of the intentions and best precautions of their managers" (p. vii).

Rosen, Clark, and Kivitz (1977) observed ways in which relatively recent court decisions had helped the 1970s reformers. They identified several portions of the *Education for All Handicapped Children Act* that had been influenced by judicial decisions.

> Early in this decade, federal and state courts began to apply constitutional concepts, such as due process, protection from cruel and unusual punishment, and equal protection under the law, to mentally retarded citizens. . . . One principle that is increasingly applied is that of the "least restrictive alternative." . . . Exclusionary policies of public schools that served to deny many mentally retarded children an education were first successfully attacked in Pennsylvania. . . . In 1971, a federal court. . . . [mandated] that Pennsylvania's public schools must cease the exclusion

of mental [*sic*] retarded children. . . . Furthermore, parents must be notified of placement in a special class or school and are entitled to an independent assessment with a formal hearing for their child to determine whether that class is appropriate for him according to his abilities. (pp. 351–352)

Sales, Powell, and Van Duizend (1982) had observed the rapid and extensive educational changes of the 1970s. Wishing to explain those changes, they looked for a connection between PL 94–142 and the state special education laws that had preceded it. They noted that increasingly comprehensive state laws had been approved during the 1960s. Although they conceded that these changes indicated politically progressive attitudes, they also discerned indications of regressive attitudes. For example, the citizens and legislators in some states demonstrated regressive attitudes when they did not repeal antiquated laws that continued to oppress disabled persons. Sales, Powell, and Van Duizend railed against outdated laws that "barred from an education those deemed 'uneducable' by school officials who, for reasons of administrative convenience, ignorance or lack of funds, chose not to deal with special education students" (p. 331). Sales, Powell, and Van Duizend did concede that recent court decisions had been weakening many antiquated state laws. In fact, they thought that those court decisions had promoted "dramatic progress." Even though they recognized the ways in which court decisions had influenced the *Education of all Handicapped Children Act*, the three scholars believed that this immensely influential law was primarily the result of "advocacy on behalf of handicapped children throughout the nation" (p. 332).

Like other scholars, Scheerenberger (1987) searched for events that had prepared the way for the groundbreaking reforms of the 1970s. He concentrated his attention on the ways in which judges, state lawmakers, educational bureaucrats, federal legislators, and even presidents had formed political alliances with the advocates for special education. Scheerenberger believed that these alliances would not have developed without the pressure from disgruntled parents. The parents were upset that their educational demands had been ignored for decades. They insisted on reform.

The parents of children with disabilities did not confine their protestations to educational issues. They were angry about mandatory institutionalization and coerced sexual sterilization. They fumed over inadequate healthcare, occupational training, and social services. They objected to the ways in which governmental policies, procedures, and programs had compromised the lives of all disabled persons. Through their sustained advocacy, they changed the attitudes of professionals in healthcare, social services, and education. They eventually changed the attitudes of government leaders.

Cross (2004) proffered a distinctive explanation for the rapid and dramatic changes that had transpired during the 1970s. He believed that the congressional hearings that accompanied PL 94–142 had substantively influenced that bill's fate. Cross reported that "the stories of how children were denied services were heartrending" and "more compelling than testimony given by any official from either the states or the federal government" (p. 56). Sensitive to the broad political dynamics of that era, Cross demonstrated his insightfulness when he described ways in which the national *zeitgeist* also had benefited this legislation. Cross recollected that the *Education for All Handicapped Children Act* had "reached the White House after the Nixon resignation," a period during which President Ford's "relations with Congress were far too fragile" for him to challenge the law. Cross concluded that "there was simply no way the bill could have been vetoed in that climate" (p. 56).

During the 1970s, the passage of PL 94–142 was facilitated by the public's changing perspective toward students with disabilities. At the same time, this law, once it had been enacted, helped to change the public's perspective. The enacted law changed other aspects of society. For example, it changed the ways in which special learners in the schools were evaluated, classified, and instructed. Wishing to understand the primary source of these transformations, some scholars examined the historical movement to establish special education. They noted the ways in which this century-and-a-half-long movement had influenced schooling in Europe and the United States. They concluded that the events of the 1970s, even though they seemed to emerge spontaneously, were connected inextricably to earlier events.

Unlike those scholars who assumed a wide and extended historical viewpoint, some of them focused on the ways in which the peculiar events of the 1970s influenced special education. They carefully examined the legislation that had been enacted in the states. They also paid attention to court rulings, the activities of parent lobbyists, congressional practices, journalistic exposes, advocacy by educators, and the broad political dynamics of the decade. Sarason and Doris (1979) observed that the 1970s educational changes were connected to a larger set of contemporary political dynamics that comprised "diverse and even conflicting and contradictory tendencies" (p. ix). These two scholars reasoned philosophically that the treatment of persons with disabilities became, in the final analysis, "a function of the nature of our society and its history" (p. ix).

Effects of PL 94–142

Public Law 94–142 was signed by President Ford in 1975. It was not implemented until October, 1977. Even though the explicit provisions of this law created changes, those changes differed from region to region. Soon after the law was passed, Sarason and Doris (1979) had predicted these regional variations. For example, they had predicted differences in the way that urban, suburban, and rural school districts would implement the legislation. They identified numerous other regional factors that would contribute to uneven implementation. These other factors included "racial and ethnic composition, average achievement levels, serious problems of management and discipline, class size, frequency of families moving within a school district, teacher morale, and level of conflict between school personnel and the community" (Sarason & Doris, 1979, p. 378). The two scholars speculated that "only if we were living in another world, could one avoid predicting that the consequences . . . will very likely be different" in distinct school districts.

Some of the differences in the ways that PL 94–142 was implemented could have been attributed to state, regional, community, and school demographics. However, the law's uneven implementation also was the result of the distinct ways in which educators, parents, government bureaucrats, and judges viewed the "spirit" of the law. Sarason and Doris (1979) gave examples in which interpretations of the original law had affected student mainstreaming, which was the practice of placing children with disabilities in regular education classrooms. Although they could not identify an explicit reference to mainstreaming within PL 94–142, the advocates of this practice believed that it was implicit within the legislation. After they had documented that less restrictive environments were guaranteed by law, they stipulated that regular education classrooms were less restrictive than special education classrooms. On the basis of this logic, they concluded that PL 94–142 implicitly sanctioned mainstreaming. Needless to say, not all educators, government bureaucrats, or judges agreed with this conclusion.

Sarason and Doris (1979) were impressed by the speed with which mainstreaming had emerged as a concept and then been implemented as a practice. They wrote that this speed had been "little short of amazing" (p. 355). Many supporters of special education shared their amazement. They particularly may have been impressed because mainstreaming represented a 180-degree shift from the previous educational course that most special education supporters had been pursuing. Earlier supporters had seen the placement of disabled students in special classrooms as the ideal way to meet distinctive needs. A new generation of advocates began to view the traditional placements as instances of *de facto* segregation. Depicting themselves as proponents of civil rights, these reformers compared the children in special education classrooms to the children in racially segregated classrooms. Sarason and Doris paraphrased the rhetoric of these reformers.

> From a narrow, legalistic standpoint, it may be inappropriate to view Public Law 94–142 as an attempt at mainstreaming. But it is clearly not inappropriate to say

that the law never could have been written and passed except in a climate suffused with the mainstreaming considerations explicitly contained in the 1954 desegregation decision. If the law is being "misinterpreted" as mainstreaming legislation, it is due less to what the law actually says and more to a perception of some people that the law was a derivative of anti-segregation sentiment. (p. 370)

The federal legislators who had passed the *Education of All Handicapped Children Act* wished to monitor its impact. Therefore, they ordered the officials in the federal Department of Education to report about the effects of the law's implementation. In one of the early reports, officials assured the legislators that "the Act is working" (United States Department of Education, 1980, p. iii). The officials followed this declaration with a list of the reasons that they were sanguine.

More children than ever before are profiting from special education. More parents are directly and positively involved in their child's schooling. Every district sampled has made changes in its programs and procedures . . . New services are being provided . . . and new opportunities for participation in education programs with nonhandicapped children have been created. (p. iii)

The authors (United States Department of Education, 1980) of the preceding paragraph extolled the benefits of *Education of All Handicapped Children Act*. However, they did concede that several problems had accompanied the new law. For example, they noted that "some children are unserved, some parents are not participating," and that some schools were offering "more services than they feel they can afford" (p. iv). After they had assessed both the benefits and the problems that the legislation had produced, the federal officials remained optimistic.

This optimism is not because the national Act is the answer to all of our problems, but because it is part of a pattern of State laws in 49 States directed at the same ends, because it works in concert with Federal and State court orders . . . and, most importantly, because our experiences as well as our studies indicate that the value systems of Americans in every community support its purposes. (p. iv)

In subsequent reports (United States Department of Education, 1981; 1982; 1983; 1984), federal bureaucrats remained positive about the *Education of All Handicapped Children Act*. However, they also realized that President Reagan and his administrators had established new national educational priorities. The restraint of spending was one of these priorities. Other priorities emerged in *A Nation at Risk* (National Commission on Excellence in Education, 1983). The authors of this widely publicized report alleged that a dysfunctional educational system imperiled economic progress and national security (Giordano, 2005). They recommended academic measures to raise academic achievement and expand educational accountability.

In 1985, the staff members of the Department of Education (United States Department of Education, 1985) presented their annual report about the *Education of All Handicapped Children Act*. Although the authors of that report discussed the cumulative effects of the *Education of All Handicapped Children Act*, they explicitly reviewed some highlights from the preceding school year. They also discussed the shifting political landscape in which they found themselves. For example, they acknowledged that they were being urged to reduce the expense of special education. Responding to this adjuration, the authors wrote that they had located strategies to "simultaneously increase services and decrease costs" (p. iv).

In their 1985 report, the staff members of the Department of Education (United States Department of Education, 1985) acknowledged the intense pressure created by the recent publication of *A Nation at Risk* (National Commission on Excellence in Education, 1983). They characterized *A Nation at Risk* as "one of the most significant educational events to occur during this reporting period" (p. iv). Whereas the *Education of All Handicapped Children Act* had focused attention on educational equity, *A Nation at Risk* shifted attention to educational excellence. The Department of Education authors, who retained their personal commitment to special learners, professed that "excellence and equity are inseparable" (United States Department of Education, 1985, p. iv). Nonetheless, they realized that they had to implement the recommendations from *A Nation at Risk*. One of these recommendations was to use education to promote economic productivity. They assured members of Congress that they could stimulate the economy through special education programs. They proposed "a major initiative to improve the services available to handicapped adolescents moving from education to the world of work" (p. iv).

Summary

During the 1970s, educational analysts detected transformations in the ways that students with disabilities were being treated. Some of the analysts linked these transformations to historical initiatives. Others connected them to contemporary political events. Irrespective of their views about causes, both groups agreed that the transformations were substantive and pervasive. They also acknowledged the unprecedented speed at which the changes were transpiring. This rapid rate decreased as new educational priorities emerged during the early 1980s.

References

Abbot, E. S. (1920). Program for mental hygiene in the public schools. *Mental Hygiene, 4* (2), 320–330.

Abbott, E., & Breckenridge, S. P. (1917). *Truancy and non-attendance in the Chicago public schools.* Chicago: University of Chicago Press.

Addams, G. S. (1914). Defectives in the juvenile court. *Training School Bulletin, 11,* 49–54.

Allen, E. E. (1904). Education of defectives. *Monographs on education in the United States, 15,* 771–819.

Allison, H. E. (1904). Defective inmates of penal institutions. *Proceedings of the Annual Congress of the National Prison Association of the United States,* 292–303.

Anderson, M. L. (1917). *Education of defectives in the public schools.* New York: World.

Anderson, V. V. (1915–1916). A classification of borderline mental cases amongst offenders. *Journal of Criminal Law, Criminology and Police Science, 6,* 689–695.

Anderson, V. V. (1919). Mental defect in a southern state. *Mental Hygiene, 4,* 527–565.

Anderson, V. V. (1920). State institutions for the feeble-minded. *Mental Hygiene, 4,* 626–646.

Anderson, V. V. (1921). Education of mental defectives in state and private institutions and in special classes in public schools in the United States. *Mental Hygiene, 5,* 85–122.

Anderson, V. V., & Fearing, F. M. (1923). *A study of the careers of 322 feebleminded persons.* New York: National Committee for Mental Hygiene.

Arlidge, J. T. (1859). *On the state of lunacy and the legal provision for the insane, with observations on the construction and organization of asylums.* London: Churchill.

Arnold, G. B. (1938). A brief review of the first thousand patients eugenically sterilized at the state colony for epileptics and feebleminded. *Journal of Psycho-Asthenics, 43* (1), 56–63.

Arnold, G. B. (1939). What eugenic sterilization has meant to the Virginia state colony for epileptics and feebleminded. *Journal of Psycho-Asthenics, 44* (2), 173–177.

Arnold, J. (1936). A sterilization law for Kentucky: Its constitutionality. *Kentucky Law Review, 24*, 220–229.

Ayres, L. P. (1911). The relative responsibility of school and society for the over-age child. *Journal of Education, 74* (24), 657–659.

Baker, B. W. (1927). Presidential address. *Journal of Psycho-Asthenics, 32*, 168–178.

Barnes, E. (1908). The public school and the special child. *National Education Association Journal of Proceedings and Addresses of the Forty-sixth Annual Meeting*, 1118–1123.

Barr, M. W. (1899–1900). The how, the why, and the wherefore of the training of feeble-minded children. *Journal of Psycho-Asthenics, 4*, 204–212.

Barr, M. W. (1902). The imbecile and the epileptic versus the tax-payer and the community. *Proceedings of the National Conference of Charities and Correction at the Twenty-Ninth Annual Session*, 161–164.

Barr, M. W. (1904). *Mental defectives: Their history, treatment and training*. Philadelphia: Blackiston's Son.

Barrows, S. J. (1888). Discussion of the provision for the feeble-minded. *Proceedings of the National Conference of Charities and Correction at the Fifteenth Annual Session*, 394–403.

Bernstein, C. (1917). Discussion. *Journal of Sociologic Medicine, 18* (3), 201–210.

Bernstein, C. (1918). Self-sustaining feeble-minded. *Journal of Psycho-Asthenics, 22* (1), 150–161.

Bernstein, C. (1920). Colony and extra-institutional care for the feebleminded. *Mental Hygiene, 4*, 1–28.

Bernstein, C. (1923). Colony and parole care for dependents and defectives. *Mental Hygiene, 7*, 449–471.

Berry, C. (1923). The mentally retarded child in the public schools. *Mental Hygiene, 7*, 762–769.

Berry, D. (1909). Mentally defective children in school and afterwards. *Journal of the Royal Institute of Public Health, 17*, 331–341.

Best, H. (1930). A comparison of the educational treatment of the deaf, the blind, and the feeble-minded. *American Journal of Sociology, 35*, 631–639.

Bevis, W. M. (1918). Colony care for the epileptic and feeble-minded of Florida. *Journal of the Florida Medical Association, 4* (11), 322–325.

Bicknell, G. H. (1907). The influence of defective sight and hearing on mental development. *Journal of Psycho-Asthenics, 11*, 27–30.

Binet, A., & Simon, T. (1914). *Mentally defective children* (W.B. Drummond, Trans.). New York: Longmans, Green.

Blatt, B. (1973). *Souls in extremis: An anthology on victims and victimizers*. Boston: Allyn & Bacon.

Blatt, B. (1981). *In and out of mental retardation*. Baltimore: University Park Press.

Blatt, B., & Kaplan, F. (1966). *Christmas in purgatory: A photographic essay on mental retardation*. Boston: Allyn & Bacon.

Bolton, F. E. (1912). Public education of exceptional children. *Educational Review, 44*, 62–69.

Bowers, P. E. (1917). The necessity for medical examination of prisoners at the time of trial. *Journal of Sociologic Medicine, 18* (3), 221–233.

Brace, C. L. (1857). *Address upon the industrial school movement.* New York: Wynkoop, Hallenbeck & Thomas.

Brace, C. L. (1859). *The best method of disposing of our pauper and vagrant children.* New York: Wynkoop, Hallenbeck & Thomas.

Braddock, D. (1987). *Federal policy toward mental retardation and developmental disabilities.* Baltimore, MD: Brookes.

Bridgman, O. (1930). An experimental study of abnormal children, with special reference to the problems of dependency and delinquency. In W. Brown, G. M. Stratton, & E. C. Tolman (Eds.), *University of California Publications in Psychology* (Volume III, pp. 1–59). Berkeley, CA: University of California Press.

Brigham, A. (1845). Schools in lunatic asylums. *American Journal of Insanity, 2,* 284–288.

Brigham, A. (1847). The moral treatment of insanity. *American Journal of Insanity, 4,* 1–15.

Brigham, A. (1848). Schools and asylums for the idiotic and imbecile. *American Journal of Insanity, 5,* 19–33.

Brockett, L. P. (1855). Idiots and institutions for their training. *American Journal of Education, 1,* 593–608.

Bronner, A. F. (1916). What do psychiatrists mean? *Journal of Mental of Nervous Disease, 44,* 30–33.

Bronner, A. F. (1923). *The psychology of special abilities and disabilities.* Boston: Little, Brown.

Brown, G. (1889). Public aid for the feeble-minded. *Proceedings of the National Conference of Charities and Correction at the Sixteenth Annual Conference,* 86–88.

Bucknill, J. C., & Tuke, D. H. (1968). *A manual of psychological medicine.* New York: Hafner-Douglas.

Bullard, W. N. (1910). The high-grade mental defectives. *Journal of Psycho-Asthenics, 14,* 14–15.

Bulter, A. W. (1907). The burden of feeble-mindedness. *Proceedings of the National Conference of Charities and Correction at the Thirty-Fourth Annual Session,* 1–10.

Burk, C. F. (1900). Promotion of bright and slow children. *Educational Review, 19,* 296–302.

Campbell, C. M. (1917a). Educational methods and the fundamental causes of dependency. *Mental Hygiene, 1* (2), 235–240.

Carson, J. C. (1899). Prevention of feeble-mindedness from a moral and legal standpoint. *Proceedings of the National Conference of Charities and Correction at the Twenty-Fifth Annual Session,* 294–303.

Chace, L. G. (1903). The education of mentally deficient children in special day classes. *Charities, 11,* 385–394.

Chace, L. G. (1904). Public school classes for mentally deficient children. *Proceedings of the National Conference of Charities and Correction at the Thirty-First Annual Session,* 390–401.

Churchill, F. (1851a). On the mental disorders of pregnancy and childbed [Part 1]. *American Journal of Insanity, 7,* 259–266.

Churchill, F. (1851b). On the mental disorders of pregnancy and childbed [Part 2]. *American Journal of Insanity, 7,* 296–317.

Clarke, W. (1915). Prostitution and mental deficiency. *Journal of Social Hygiene, 1,* 364–387.

Classic articles in special education: Articles that shaped the field, 1960 to 1996 (2004). *Remedial and Special Education, 25* (2), 79–87.

Claxton, P. P. (1911). Letter of transmittal. In J. H. Van Sickle, L. Witmer, & L. P. Ayres, *Provision for Exceptional Children in Public Schools* (USBE No. 14, p. 5). Washington, DC: Government Printing Office.

Collar, G., & Crook, C. H. (1905). *School management and methods of instruction with special reference to elementary schools.* New York: Macmillan. (Original work published in 1900)

Connolly, J. (1846). Imbecility of mind supervening in young people. *American Journal of Insanity, 3,* 141–145.

Conolly, J. (1850). Diversities of human character, and delicate shades of insanity, their relation to offences and crimes. *American Journal of Insanity, 6,* 289–307.

Cornell, E. L., & Ross, E. (1928). Principles underlying special class organization in New York State. *Training School Bulletin, 25,* 81–96.

Cornell, W. B. (1921). The organization of state institutions for feeble-minded in the United States. *Journal of Psycho-Asthenics, 25,* 21–27.

Crafts, L. W. (1916–1917). A bibliography on the relation of crime and feeble-mindedness. *Journal of Criminal Law and Criminology, 7,* 544–554.

Cronin, J. M. (1976). The federal takeover: Should junior partner run the firm? *Phi Delta Kappan, 57,* 499–501.

Cross, C. T. (2004). *Political education: national policy comes of age.* New York: Teachers College Press.

Crowley, R. H. (1910). *The hygiene of school life.* London: Methuen & Company.

Curtis, H. (1924). The iron man and the feeble-minded. *School and Society, 19,* 643–644.

Davenport, A. B. (1920). Selecting immigrants. *Journal of Psycho-Asthenics, 25,* 178–179.

Davenport, C. B. (1911). A census of the feeble-minded in institutions and poorhouses. *Journal of Psycho-Asthenics, 16* (1), 9–11.

Davies, S. P. (1923). *Social control of the feebleminded: A study of social programs and attitudes in relation to the problems of mental deficiency.* New York: National Committee for Mental Hygiene.

Dawson, G. E. (1909). A characterization of the prevailing defects in backward children and a method of studying and helping them. *Pedagogical Seminary, 16* (4), 429–436.

De Sanctis, S. (1911). Mental development and the measurement of the level of intelligence. *Journal of Educational Psychology, 2,* 498–507.

Dealey, C. E. (1923). Problem children in the early grade schools. *Journal of Abnormal Psychology and Social Psychology, 18* (2), 125–136.

DeFelice, M. G. (1851). Notice of the cretins of Switzerland, and the attempts by Dr. Guggenbuhl to educate them. *American Journal of Insanity, 7*, 235–242.

Descoeudres, A. (1928). *The education of mentally defective children: Psychological observations and practical suggestions* (E. F. Row, Trans., 2nd ed.). London: Harrap.

Devereux, H. T. (1909). Report of a year's work on defectives in a public school. *Psychological Clinic, 3*, 45–48.

Doll, E. A. (1917). *Clinical studies in feeble-mindedness.* Boston: Badger.

Doll, E. A. (1919). The problem of the mental defective. *School and Society, 10*, 187–191.

Doll, E. A. (1928). The next ten years in special education. *Training School Bulletin, 25*, 145–153.

Donkin, H. B. (1911). Introductory note. In E. B. Sherlock, *The feeble-minded: A guide to study and practice* (pp. xvii–xx). London: Macmillan.

Douglas, P. H. (1921). American apprenticeship and industrial education. *Columbia University Studies in History, Economics, and Public Law, 95* (2, Serial No. 216). (Original work published in 1918)

Down, J. L. (1876). *On the education and training of the feeble in mind.* London: Lewis.

Draper, W. F. (1919). The detention and treatment of infected women as a measure of control of venereal diseases in extra cantonment zones. *American Journal of Obstetrics and Diseases of Women and Children, 80*, 642–646.

Duncan, P. M. (1866). *A manual for the classification, training, and education of the feeble-minded, imbecile, & idiotic.* London: Longmans, Green.

Dunlop, O. J. (1912). *English apprenticeship & child labor.* New York: Macmillan.

Dunphy, M. C. (1908). Modern ideals of education applied to the training of mental defectives. *Proceedings of the National Conference on Charities and Correction at the Thirty-Fourth Annual Session*, 325–333.

East, N. (1923). Delinquency and mental defect (I). *British Journal of Medical Psychology, 3*, 153–167.

Eaton, J. J. (1917). *Record forms for vocational schools.* New York: World Book Company.

Edson, A. W. (1906–1907). Special plans for the promotion of backward pupils. *Kindergarten Magazine and Pedagogical Digest, 19*, 397–403.

Edson, A. W. (1908). The education in public schools of the deaf, cripples and mental defectives. *Education, 28*, 351–355.

Education for All Handicapped Children Act, PL 94–142. (1975). Retrieved from http://thomas.loc.gov/bss

Edwards, N. (1933). *The courts and the public schools.* Chicago: University of Chicago Press.

Eliot, T. D. (1925). Welfare agencies, special education, and the courts. *American Journal of Sociology, 3*, 58–78.

Erikson, M. H. (1931). Some aspects of abandonment, feeblemindedness, and crime. *American Journal of Sociology, 36*, 758–769.

Farrell, E. E. (1908a). Special classes in New York City schools. *Journal for Psycho-Asthenics, 13* (1), 91–96.

Farrell, E. E. (1908b). The problems of the special class. *National Education Association of the United States Proceedings and Addresses*, 1131–1136.

Farrell, E. E. (1908–1909). Special classes in the New York City schools. *Journal of Psycho-Asthenics, 13*, 91–96.

Farrell, E. E. (1914a). A study of the school inquiry report on ungraded classes [*Part I*]. *Psychological Clinic, 8* (2), 29–47.

Farrell, E. E. (1914b). A study of the school inquiry report on ungraded classes [*Part II*]. *Psychological Clinic, 8* (3), 57–74.

Farrell, E. E. (1914c). A study of the school inquiry report on ungraded classes [*Part III*]. *Psychological Clinic, 8* (4), 99–106.

Farrell, E. E. (1914d). Introduction. In B. S. Morgan, *The backward child: A study of the psychology and treatment of backwardness* (pp. iii–vii). New York: Putnam's Sons.

Fernald, G. G. (1912). The defective delinquent class differentiating tests. *American Journal of Insanity, 68* (4), 523–594.

Fernald, G. G. (1920). Curative treatment vs. punishment for defective delinquents. *Journal of Psycho-Asthenics, 25*, 161–167.

Fernald, W. E. (1893). The history of the treatment of the feeble-minded. *Proceedings of the National Conference of Charities and Correction at the Twentieth Annual Session, 20*, 203–221.

Fernald, W. E. (1909). The imbecile with criminal instincts. *Journal of Psycho-Asthenics, 14* (1), 16–38.

Fernald, W. E. (1912). The burden of the feeble-mindedness. *Journal of Psycho-Asthenics, 17*, 18–111.

Fernald, W. E. (1917). The growth of provision for the feeble-minded in the United States. *Journal of Mental Hygiene, 1*, 34–59.

Fernald, W. E. (1918). Some of the limitations of the plan for segregation of the feeble-minded. *Ungraded, 3*, 171–176.

Fernald, W. E. (1919). A state program for the care of mentally defective. *Mental Hygiene, 3*, 566–574.

Fernald, W. E. (1923). The subnormal child. *School and Society, 18*, 397–406.

Findlay, J. J. (1911). *Principles of class teaching*. London: Macmillan.

Fitts, A. M. (1916). How to fill the gap between special classes and institutions. *Journal of Psycho-Asthenics, 21*, 79–87.

Fitts, A. M. (1920). The value of special classes for the mentally defective pupils in the public schools. *Journal of Psycho-Asthenics, 25*, 114–123.

Foster, W. W. (1909, November). Hereditary criminality and its certain cure. *Pearson's Magazine, 22* (5), 565–572.

Frampton, M. E., & Gall, E. D. (Eds.). (1955a). *Special education for the exceptional: Vol. 1. Introduction and problems*. Boston: Sargent.

Frampton, M. E., & Gall, E. D. (Eds.). (1955b). *Special education for the exceptional: Vol. 2—The physically handicapped and special health problems*. Boston: Sargent.

Frampton, M. E., & Gall, E. D. (Eds.). (1956). *Special education for the exceptional: Vol. 3. Mental and emotional deviates and special problems.* Boston: Sargent.

Frampton, M. E., & Rowell, H. G. (Eds.). (1938). *Education of the handicapped: Vol. 1. History.* New York: World.

Franz, S. I. (1912). *Handbook of mental examination methods* (Nervous and Mental Disease Monograph Series No. 10). New York: Journal of Nervous and Mental Disease Publishing Company.

Gardner, D. C., & Warren S. A. (1978). Careers and disabilities: A career education approach. Stamford, CT: Greylock.

Gegenheimer, R. A. (1948). A quarter century of community supervision of mentally deficient patients. *American Journal of Mental Deficiency, 53* (1), 93–102.

Gesell, A. (1913, October). The village of a thousand souls. *American Magazine, 76* (4), 11–15.

Gesell, A. (1921). *Exceptional children and public school policy: Including a mental survey of the New Haven elementary schools.* New Haven, CT: Yale University Press.

Getz, C., & Kelley, W. M. (1956). Problems relating to children born out of wedlock. In M. E. Frampton & E. D. Gall (Eds.), *Special education for the exceptional: Vol. 3. Mental and emotional deviates and special problems* (pp. 346–353). Boston: Sargent.

Gilbert, C. B. (1906). *The school and its life.* New York: Silver, Burdett.

Giordano, G. (2000). *Twentieth-century reading education: The era of remedial reading.* New York, NY: Elsevier.

Giordano, G. (2003). *Twentieth-century textbook wars: A history of advocacy and opposition.* New York: Peter Lang.

Giordano, G. (2004). *Wartime schools: How World War II changed American education.* New York: Peter Lang.

Giordano, G. (2005). *How testing came to dominate American schools: The history of educational assessment.* New York: Peter Lang.

Goddard, H. H. (1912). The improvability of feeble-minded children. *Journal of Psycho-Asthenics, 16,* 119–131.

Goddard, H. H. (1914). *Feeble-mindedness: Its causes and consequences.* New York: Macmillan.

Goddard, H. H. (1917). Introduction. In M. L. Anderson. *Education of defectives in the public schools* (pp. ix–xvii). New York: World.

Goddard, H. H. (1923). *School training of defective children* (4th ed.). New York: World.

Goldney, R. D., & Schioldann, J. A. (2002). *Pre-Durkheim suicidology: The 1892 reviews of Tuke and Savage.* Australia: Adelaide.

Green, J. A. (1911). A note on backward children. *Journal of Experimental Pedagogy and Training College Record, 1* (2), 158–159.

Green, J. A. (1912). A note on backward children. *Journal of Experimental Pedagogy and Training College Record, 1* (3), 223–226.

Greene, H. M. (1884). The obligation of civilized society to idiotic and feeble-minded children. *Proceedings of the National Conference of Charities and Corrections at the Eleventh Annual Meeting,* 264–271.

Greenwell, D. (1869). *On the education of the imbecile.* London: Strahan.

Groszmann, M. P. E. (1907). Some phases of eccentric mentality in children. *Education, 28,* 90–96.

Groszmann, M. P. E. (1913). A tentative classification of exceptional children. *Child, 4,* 33–39.

Groszmann, M. P. E. (1917a). Some recent changes in the attitude towards the problem of mental defect. *Educational Foundations, 29* (1), 24–29.

Groszmann, M. P. E. (1917b). *The exceptional child.* New York: Scribner's Sons.

Groszmann, W. H. (1906). The position of the atypical child. *Journal of Nervous and Mental Disease, 33* (7), 425–446.

Haber, R. (1917). Introduction. In S. W. Hamilton & R. Haber, *Summaries of state laws relating to the feebleminded and the epileptic* (pp. vii–ix). New York: National Committee for Mental Hygiene.

Hall, G. S. (1914). Introduction. In J. E. W. Wallin, *The mental health of the school child (pp. xvii–xix).* New Haven: Yale University Press. (Original work published in 1901)

Hamilton, L. (1906). Education of the backward child. *Educational Work, 1,* 6–7.

Hamilton, S. W., & Haber, R. (1917). *Summaries of state laws relating to the feebleminded and the epileptic.* New York: National Committee for Mental Hygiene.

Hanus, P. H. (1913). *School efficiency: A constructive study applied to New York City.* New York: World.

Hardy, I. (1913). Schools for the feeble-minded state's best insurance policy. *Southern Medical Journal, 6,* 511–516.

Hart, H. H. (1910). *Preventative treatment of neglected children.* New York: Charities Publication Committee.

Harvey, T. E. (1913). Preface. In J. Wormwald & S. Wormwald, *A guide to the Mental Deficiency Act, 1913* (pp. vii–x). London: King & Son.

Henderson, C. R. (1901). *Introduction to the study of the dependent, defective, and delinquent classes and their social treatment.* Boston: Heath. (Original work published in 1893)

Hill, A. S. (1957). *The forward look: The severely retarded child goes to school.* Washington, DC: United Sates Government Printing Office. (Original work published in 1952)

Hinshelwood, J. (1900). Congenital word-blindness. *Lancet, 1,* 1506–1508.

Hinshelwood, J. (1917). *Congenital word-blindness.* London: Lewis.

Hoffman, E. (1975). The American public school and the deviant child: The origins of their involvement. *Journal of Special Education, 9* (4), 416–423.

Hollingworth, L. S. (1922). Differential action upon the sexes of forces which tend to segregate the feeble-minded. *Journal of Abnormal Psychology and Social Psychology, 17* (1), 35–57.

Hollingworth, L. S. (1923). *Special talents and defects: Their significance for education.* New York: Macmillan.

Holmes, A. (1911). The purpose and organization of the special class. In L. Witmer, *The special class for backward children* (pp. 11–32). Philadelphia: Psychological Clinic Press.

Holmes, A. (1912). *The conservation of the child: A manual of clinical psychology presenting the examination and treatment of backward children: A book for school executives and teachers, being an exposition of plans that have been evolved to adapt school organization to the needs of individual children.* Philadelphia: Lippincott.

Holmes, A. (1915). *Backward children.* Indianapolis, IN: Bobbs-Merrill.

Holmes, W. H. (1912). *School organization and the individual child.* Massachusetts: Davis.

Howe, S. G. (1851). On the training and educating idiots: The second annual report made to the legislature of Massachusetts. *American Journal of Insanity, 8,* 97–118.

Howe, S. G. (1852). *Third and final report of the experimental school for teaching and training idiotic children; also, the first report of the trustees of the Massachusetts school for idiotic and feeble-minded youth.* Boston: Dutton & Wentworth.

Howe, S. G. (1972). *On the causes of idiocy.* New York: Arno. (Original work published in 1848.)

Inskeep, A. D. (1926). *Teaching dull and retarded children.* New York: Macmillan.

Inskeep, A. D. (1930). *Child adjustment: In relation to growth and development.* New York: Appleton.

Ireland, W. W. (1877). *On idiocy and imbecility.* London: Churchill.

Ireland, W. W. (1898). *The mental affections of children, idiocy, imbecility and insanity.* London: Churchill.

Jarvis, E. (1852). On the supposed increase of insanity. *American Journal of Insanity, 8,* 333–364.

Jennings, H. M., & Hallock, A. L. (1913). Binet–Simon test at the George Junior Republic. *Journal of Educational Psychology, 4,* 471–475.

Johnson, A. (1898). Concerning a form of degeneracy, I: The condition and increase of the feeble-minded. *American Journal of Sociology, 4,* 326–334.

Johnson, A. (1899). Concerning a form of degeneracy, II: The education and care of the feeble-minded. *American Journal of Sociology, 4,* 463–473.

Johnstone, E. R. (1898). What we do, and how we do it. *Journal of Psycho-Asthenics, 2,* 98–105.

Johnstone, E. R. (1908). The functions of the special class. *National Education Association Journal of Proceedings and Addresses of the Forty-Sixth Annual Meeting,* 1114–1118.

Johnstone, E. R. (1909a). The summer school for teachers of backward children. *Journal of Psycho-Asthenics, 14,* 122–130.

Johnstone, E. R. (1909b). The welfare of feeble-minded children. *Pedagogical Seminary, 16,* 447–449.

Johnstone, E. R. (1916). Committee report: Stimulating public interest in the feeble-minded. *Proceedings of the National Conference on Charities and Correction at the Forty third Annual Session,* 205–215.

Jones, K. B. (1936). Discussion. *American Journal of Psychiatry, 94,* 1031–1033.

Kanner, L. (1938). Habeas corpus releases of feebleminded persons and their consequences. *American Journal of Psychiatry, 94,* 1013–1033.

Keesecker, W. W. (1933). To save the schools. *School Life, 19,* 67, 79.

Kerlin, I. N. (1877). The organization of establishments for the idiotic and imbecile classes. *Proceedings of the Association of Medical Officers of American Institutions for Idiotic and Feebleminded Persons*, 19–35.

Kerlin, I. N. (1885). Provision for idiotic and feeble-minded children. *Proceedings of the National Conference of Charities and Correction at the Eleventh Annual Session*, 246–263.

Kerlin, I. N., & Greene, H. M. (1884). *Idiotic and feebleminded children: Report of the standing committee to the eleventh national conference of charities and reforms, St. Louis, 1884*. Boston: Ellis.

Kirby, A. H. P. (1914). *Legislation for the feeble-minded*. London: John Bale, Sons & Danielsson.

Kirk, S., A., Karnes, M. B., & Kirk, W. D. (1955). *You and your retarded child: A manual for parents of retarded children*. New York: Macmillan.

Kirk, S. A., Karnes, M. B., & Kirk, W. D. (1968). *You and your retarded child: A manual for parents of retarded children* (2nd ed.). Palo Alto, CA: Pacific Books.

Kirp, D., Buss, W., & Kuriloff, P. (1974). Legal reform and special education: Empirical studies and procedural proposals. *California Law Review, 62* (1), 40–155.

Kohs, S. C. (1915–1916). Who is feeble-minded? *Journal of Criminal Law and Criminology, 6*, 860–871.

Kohs, S. C. (1916). The borderlines of mental deficiency. Journal of Psycho-Asthenics, 21, 88–103.

Kolstoe, O. P. (1972). Programs for the mildly retarded: A reply to critics. *Exceptional Children, 39* (1), 51–56.

Kuhlmann, F. (1904). Experimental studies in mental deficiency: Three cases of imbecility (Mongolian) and six cases of feeblemindedness. *American Journal of Psychology, 15*, 391–446.

Kuhlmann, F. (1915). What constitutes feeble-mindedness? *Journal of Psycho-Asthenics, 19* (4), 215–236.

Lapage, C. P. (1911). *Feeblemindedness in children of school age*. Manchester: Manchester University Press.

Lawrence, C. M. (1900). Principles of education for the feeble-minded. *Journal of Psycho-Asthenics, 31*, 100–108.

Lazerson, M., & Grubb, W. N. (Eds.). (1974). *American education and vocationalism*. New York: Teachers College Press.

Lewis, O. F. (1912–1913). The feeble-minded delinquent. *Journal of Criminal Law and Criminology, 3*, 10–11.

Lincoln, D. F. (1903). Special classes for feeble-minded children in the Boston public schools. *Journal of Psycho-Asthenics, 7*, 83–93.

MacMurchy, H. (1915). *Organization and management of auxiliary classes*. Ontario, Canada: Cameron.

MacMurchy, H. (1920). *The almosts [sic]: A study of the feeble-minded*. Boston: Houghton Mifflin Company.

Maennel, B. (1909). *Auxiliary education: The training of backward children* (E. Sylvester, Trans.). New York: Doubleday, Page.

Mann, H., Taft, B., & Calhoun, W.B. (1832). *Report of the commissioners appointed to super-intend the erection of a lunatic hospital at Worcester.* Boston: Dutton & Wentworth.

Mateer, F. (1924). *The unstable child.* New York: Appleton.

Mead, H. M. (1918). An experiment in after care work. *Ungraded, 3,* 177–183.

Merrill, M. A. (1918). The ability of the special class children in the "three R's." *Pedagogical Seminary, 25,* 88–96.

Mertz, P. (1919). Mental deficiency of prostitutes: A study of delinquent women at an army port of embarkation. *Journal of the American Medical Association, 72,* 1597–1599.

Mesibov, G. B. (1976). Mentally retarded people: 200 years in America. *Journal of Clinical Child Psychology, 5* (3), 25–29.

Milburn, R. (1908). Problems of feeble-mindedness. *Journal of Psycho-Asthenics, 13* (1), 51–73.

Millis, H. A. (1898). The law relating to the relief and care of dependents, V: The law relating to the care and treatment of the defective. *American Journal of Sociology, 4,* 51–68.

Morgan, B. S. (1914). *The backward child: A study of the psychology and treatment of back-wardness.* New York: Putnam's Sons.

Morgan, W. P. (1896). A case of congenital word blindness. *British Medical Journal, 2,* 1378.

Murchison, C. (1926). *Criminal Intelligence.* Worcester, MA: Clark University Press.

Nash, A. M., & Porteus, S. D. (1919). *Educational treatment of defectives* (Training School Bulletin No. 18). Vineland, NJ: Vineland Training School.

National Commission on Excellence in Education. (1983). *A nation at risk: The impera-tive for educational reform.* Washington, DC: Author.

Newman, M. V. (1908). Backward children—Some experiences and suggestions. *Western Journal of Education, 13,* 513–516.

Noll, S. (1995). *Feeble-minded in our midst: Institutions for the mentally retarded in the South, 1900–1940.* Chapel Hill: University of North Carolina Press.

Norsworthy, N. (1906). *The psychology of mentally deficient children.* New York: Science Press.

O'Shea, M. V. (1915). Editor's Introduction. In A. Holmes, *Backward children* (pp. 1–3). Indianapolis, IN: Bobbs-Merrill.

O'Shea, M. V. (1923). Editor's Introduction. In L. S. Hollingsworth, *Special talents and defects: Their significance for education* (pp. iii–xviii). New York: Macmillan.

Osgood, R. L. (2000). *For "children who vary from the normal type": Special education in Boston, 1838–1930.* Washington, DC: Gallaudet University Press.

Otis, E. O. (1917). The physically defective. *Journal of Sociologic Medicine, 18* (3), 191–210.

Otis, M. (1913). Binet tests applied to delinquent girls. *Psychological Clinic, 7,* 127–134.

Peterson, F. (1896). The psychology of the idiot. *American Journal of Insanity, 53,* 1–15.

Polglase, W. A. (1901). The evolution of the care of the feeble-minded and epileptic in the past century. *Proceedings of the National Conference of Charities and Correction at the Twenty-eighth Annual Session,* 186–190.

Pollock, H. M., & Furbush, E. M. (1917). Insane, feebleminded, epileptics, and ine-briates in institutions in the United States, January 1, 1917. *Mental Hygiene, 1,* 548–566.

Porteus, S. D. (1920). A plan for the study of mental defectives. *Journal of Psycho-Asthenics, 25,* 58–70.

Powell, F. M. (1887). The care and training of feeble-minded children. *Proceedings of the National Conference of Charities and Correction at the Fourteenth Annual Session,* 250–260.

Pressey, S. L., & Pressey, L. C. (1928). *Mental abnormality and deficiency: An introduction to the study of problems of mental health.* New York: Macmillan.

Pyle, W. H. (1913). Standards of mental efficiency. *Journal of Educational Psychology, 4,* 61–70.

Pyle, W. H. (1914). A study of delinquent girls. *Psychological Clinic, 8* (5), 143–149.

Randall, C. D. (1896). The Michigan system of child saving. *American Journal of Sociology, 1,* 710–724.

Ray, I. (1846). Observations on the principal hospitals for the insane, in Great Britain, France and Germany. *American Journal of Insanity, 2,* 289–390.

Ray, I. (1852). The popular feeling towards hospitals for the insane. *American Journal of Insanity, 9,* 36–65.

Reed, W. O., & Jones, G. (1957). Foreword. In A. S. Hill, *The forward look: The severely retarded child goes to school* (pp. iii–iv). Washington, DC: United Sates Government Printing Office. (Original work published in 1952.)

Renz, E. (1914). A study of the intelligence of delinquents and eugenic significance of mental defect. *Training School Bulletin, 11,* 37–42.

Richards, J. B. (1884). The education of the feeble-minded. *Proceedings of the Association of Medical Officers of American Institutions for Idiotic and Feebleminded Persons,* 419–422.

Richman, J. (1907). Special classes and special schools for delinquent and backward children. *Proceedings of the National Conference of Charities and Correction at the Thirty-Fourth Annual Session,* 232–250.

Risley, S. D. (1905). Is asexualization ever justifiable in the case of imbecile children? *Journal of Psycho-Asthenics, 9* (4), 92–98.

Rivera, G. (1972). *Willowbrook.* New York: Random House.

Rogers, A. C. (1888). Functions of a school for feeble-minded. *Proceedings of the National Conference of Charities and Correction at the Fifteenth Annual Session,* 100–106.

Rogers, A. C. (1898). Does the education of the feeble-minded pay? *Journal of Psycho-Asthenics, 2* (4), 152–154.

Rogers, A. C. (1907). Borderland cases. *Journal of Psycho-Asthenics, 11,* 19–24.

Rogers, A. C. (1912). Classification of the feeble-minded based on mental age. *Bulletin of the American Academy of Medicine, 13* (3), 135–144.

Rosen, M., Clark, G. R., & Kivitz, M. S. (1977). *Habilitation of the handicapped: New dimensions in programs for the developmentally disabled.* Baltimore, MD: University Park Press.

Rosenfeld, J. (1906). Special classes in the public schools of New York. *Education, 28,* 92–100.

Safford, P. L., & Safford, E. J. (1996). *A history of childhood and disability.* New York: Teachers College Press.

Sage, D., & Burrello, L. C. (1986). *Policy and management in special education.* Englewood Cliffs, NJ: Prentice-Hall.

Sales, B. D., Powell, D. M., and Duizend, R. V. (1982). *Disabled persons and the law: State legislative issues.* New York: Plenum.

Salisbury, A. (1892). The education of the feeble-minded. *Proceedings of the Association of Medical Officers of American Institutions for Idiotic and Feeble-Minded Persons,* 219–233.

Sarason, S. B., & Doris, J. (1979). *Educational handicap, public policy, and social history.* New York: Free Press.

Saveth, E. N. (1952, April). What historians teach about business. *Fortune* (45), 118–119, 165–174.

Scheerenberger, R. C. (1987). A history of mental retardation: *A quarter century of promise.* Baltimore, MD: Brookes.

Scheidemann, N. V. (1931). *The psychology of exceptional children: Vol. 1.* Boston: Houghton Mifflin.

Schlapp, M. G. (1915). Recent progress in dealing with feeble-minded and mentally defective dependent children. *Journal of Psycho-Asthenics, 19,* 175–186.

Scott, I. J. (1899). Report of the vacation school for the feeble-minded. *Journal of Psycho-Asthenics, 4,* 65–67.

Search, P. W. (1905). *An ideal school or, looking forward.* New York: Appleton.

Seguin, E. (1870). *New facts and remarks concerning idiocy, being a lecture delivered before the New York Medical Journal Association, October 15, 1869.* New York: Wood.

Seguin, E. (1878). Recent progress in the training of idiots. *Proceedings of the Association of Medical Officers of American Institutions for Idiotic and Feebleminded Persons,* 60–65.

Seguin, E. (1907). *Idiocy: And its treatment by the physiological method.* New York: Columbia University Press. (Original work published in 1866)

Sherlock, E. B. (1911). *The feeble-minded: A guide to study and practice.* London: Macmillan.

Sherman, E. B. (1908). What the regular class teacher should know of mental and moral deficiency. *National Education Association Journal of Proceedings and Addresses of the Forty-sixth Annual Meeting,* 943–948.

Shuttleworth, G. E. (1899). The elementary education of defective children by "special classes" in London. *Journal of Psycho-Asthenics, 4,* 58–64.

Shuttleworth, G. E., & Potts, W. A. (1922). *Mentally defective children, their treatment and training.* Philadelphia: Blakiston's Son.

Sigmon, S. B. (1987). *Radical analysis of special education: Focus on historical developmental and learning disabilities.* London: Falmer.

Smart, I. T. (1908). Some urgent needs for advancement in the education of the mentally defective children. *National Education Association Journal of Proceedings and Addresses of the Forty-sixth Annual Meeting,* 1143–1151.

Snedden, D. S. (1907). *Administration and educational work of American juvenile reform schools*. New York: Teachers College, Columbia University Press.

Spaulding, F. E. (1920). Some administrative aspects of the care of the feeble-minded in the public school system. *Journal of Psycho-Asthenics, 25*, 71–80.

Stewart, J. Q. A. (1882). The industrial department of the Kentucky institution for the education and training of feeble-minded children. *Proceedings of the Association of Medical Officers of American Institutions for Idiotic and Feeble-minded Persons*, 236–239.

Sunne, D. (1917). A comparative study of white and Negro children. *Journal of Applied Psychology, 1*, 71–83.

Talbot, E. S. (1898). *Degeneracy: Its causes, signs, and results*. London: Scott.

Taliaferro, J. C. (1930). *Vocational guidance for feebleminded children*. Unpublished master's thesis, George Washington University, Washington, DC.

Taylor, J. M. (1906). Difficult boys. *Popular Science Monthly, 69*, 338–351.

Terman, L. M. (1912). A survey of mentally defective children in the schools of San Luis Obispo, California. *Psychological Clinic, 6*, 131–139.

Terman, L. M. (1916). *The measurement of intelligence: An explanation of and a complete guide for the use of the Stanford revision and extension of the Binet-Simon intelligence scale*. Boston: Houghton Mifflin.

Terman, L. M. (1917). Feeble-minded children in the public schools of California. *School and Society, 5*, 161–165.

Thomas, C. J. (1905). Congenital "word-blindness" and its treatment. *Ophthalmoscope, 3*, 380–385.

Town, C. H., & Hill, G. E. (n.d.). *How the feebleminded live in the community: A report of a social investigation of the Erie County feebleminded discharged from the Rome state school, 1905–1924*. Buffalo, NY: Children's Aid Society.

Tozier, J. (1911a, May). An educational wonder-worker: The methods of Maria Montessori. *McClure's Magazine, 37* (1), 3–19.

Tozier, J. (1911b, December). The Montessori schools in Rome: The revolutionary educational work of Maria Montessori as carried out in her own schools. *McClure's Magazine, 38* (2), 123–137.

Tozier, J. (1912, January). The Montessori apparatus: A description of the material and apparatus used in teaching by the Montessori Method. *McClure's Magazine, 38* (3), 289–302.

Tredgold, A. F. (1908). *Mental Deficiency*. New York: William Wood.

Trent, J. W. (1998). Defectives at the world's fair: Constructing disability in 1904. *Remedial and Special Education, 19*, 201–211.

Tuke, D. H. (1872). *Illustrations of the influence of the mind upon the body in health and disease, designed to elucidate the action of the imagination*. Philadelphia: Lea's Son.

Tuke, D. H. (1875). *On the Richmond asylum schools*. Lewes: G. P. Bacon. (Reprinted from *Journal of Mental Science*, October, 1875)

Tuke, D. H. (1878). *Insanity in ancient modern life, with chapters on its prevention*. London: Macmillan.

Tuke, D. H. (1882). *Chapters in the history of the insane in the British Isles.* London: Kegan, Paul & Trench.

Tuke, D. H. (1885). *The insane in the United States and Canada.* London: Lewis.

Tuke, D. H. (Ed.). (1892a). *A dictionary of psychological medicine: Vol. 1.* London: Churchill.

Tuke, D. H. (Ed.). (1892b). *A dictionary of psychological medicine: Vol. 2.* London: Churchill.

Tuke, D. H. (1892c). *Reform in the treatment of the insane—Early history of the Retreat, York: Its objects and influence, with a report of the celebrations of its centenary.* London: Churchill.

Tuke, D. H. (1894). *Alleged increase in insanity in England and Wales.* Lewes: South Counties Press. (Reprinted from *Journal of Mental Science*, April, 1894)

Tuke, J. B. (1868). Objections to the cottage system of treatment for lunatics as it now exists, and suggestions for its improvement and elaboration. *Edinburgh Medical Journal, 13* (10), 916–918.

Tuke, J. B. (1898). Modern conceptions of the etiology of the insanities. *British Medical Journal, 2* (1962), 341–344.

Tuke, S. (1815a). *A letter on pauper lunatic asylums.* New York: Samuel Wood & Sons.

Tuke, S. (1815b). *Practical hints on the construction and economy of pauper lunatic asylums: Including instructions to the architects who offered plans for the Wakefield asylum and a sketch of the most approved design.* New York: Alexander.

Tuke, S. (1964). *Description of the Retreat.* London: Dawsons. (Original work published in 1813)

United States Department of Education. (1980). *Second Annual Report to Congress on the Implementation of the Public Law 94–142: The Education for All Handicapped Children Act.* Washington, DC: Government Printing Office.

United States Department of Education. (1981). *Third Annual Report to Congress on the Implementation of the Public Law 94–142: The Education for All Handicapped Children Act.* Washington, DC: Government Printing Office.

United States Department of Education. (1982). *Fourth Annual Report to Congress on the Implementation of the Public Law 94–142: The Education for All Handicapped Children Act.* Washington, DC: Government Printing Office.

United States Department of Education. (1983). *Fifth Annual Report to Congress on the Implementation of the Public Law 94–142: The Education for All Handicapped Children Act.* Washington, DC: Government Printing Office.

United States Department of Education. (1984). *Sixth Annual Report to Congress on the Implementation of the Public Law 94–142: The Education for All Handicapped Children Act.* Washington, DC: Government Printing Office.

United States Department of Education. (1985). *Seventh Annual Report to Congress on the Implementation of the Public Law 94–142: The Education for All Handicapped Children Act.* Washington, DC: Government Printing Office.

Van Sickle, J. H., Witmer, L., & Ayres, L. P. (1911). *Provision for Exceptional Children in Public Schools* (USBE No. 14). Washington, DC: Government Printing Office.

Walker, J. (1930). Factors contributing to the delinquency of defective girls. In W. Brown, G. M. Stratton, & E. C. Tolman (Eds.), *University of California Publications in Psychology*, (Vol. III, pp. 147–213). Berkeley, CA: University of California Press.

Wallin, J. E. W. (1914). *The mental health of the school child.* New Haven: Yale University Press.

Wallin, J. E. W. (1915–1916). Who is feeble-minded? *Journal of Criminal Law, Criminology and Police Science, 6*, 706–716.

Wallin, J. E. W. (1917). Feeblemindedness and delinquency. *Mental Hygiene, 1*, 585–590.

Wallin, J. E. W. (1921a). A comparison of three methods for making the initial selection of presumptive mental defects. *School and Society, 13*, 31–45.

Wallin, J. E. W. (1921b). Suggested rules for special classes. *Educational Administration and Supervision, 7*, 447–457.

Wallin, J. E. W. (1922a). A study of the industrial record of children assigned to public school classes for mental defectives, and the legislation in the interest of defectives. *Journal of Abnormal Psychology and Social Psychology, 17* (2), 120–131.

Wallin, J. E. W. (1922b). An investigation of the sex, relationship, marriage, delinquency and truancy of children assigned to special public school classes. *Journal of Abnormal Psychology and Social Psychology, 17* (1), 19–34.

Wallin, J. E. W. (1931). The Baltimore plan of training special class teachers and other workers in the field of special education. *Elementary School Journal, 31* (8), 607–618.

Wallin, J. E. W. (1933). Check lists of supplies and equipment for special classes for mentally deficient and backward children. *Training School Bulletin, 30* (8), 145–152.

Warner, A. G. (1894). *American charities: A study in philanthropy and economics.* New York: Crowell.

Weidensall, J. (1914). Psychological tests as applied to the criminal women. *Psychological Review, 21*, 370–375.

White, W. A. (1949). Introduction. In A. Deutsch, *The mentally ill in America: A history of their care and treatment from colonial times* (2nd ed., pp. v–x). New York: Columbia University Press. (Original work published in 1938)

Wilbur, C. T. (1888). Institutions for the feeble-minded: The results of forty years of effort in establishing them in the United States. *Proceedings of the National Conference of Charities and Correction at the Fifteenth Annual Session*, 106–113.

Wilbur, H. B. (1862). Some suggestions on the principles and methods of elementary instruction. Albany, NY: Munsell.

Williams, T. A. (1909). Psychoprophylaxis in childhood. *Journal of Abnormal Psychology, 4* (2), 182–199.

Wilmarth, A. (1898). The rights of the public in dealing with defective classes. *Journal of the American Medical Association, 31*, 1276–1279.

Winzer, M. A. (1993). *The history of special education: From isolation to integration.* Washington, DC: Gallaudet University Press.

Witmer, L. (1915). The exceptional child and the training of teachers for exceptional children. *School and Society, 2*, 217–229.

Witmer, L. (1916). Congenital aphasia and feeblemindedness: A clinical diagnosis. *Psychological Clinic, 10*, 181–191.

Witmer, L. (1919, April). What I did with Don. *Ladies' Home Journal*, pp. 51, 122–123.

Woodrow, H. (1919). *Brightness and dullness in children*. Philadelphia: Lippincott.

Woodrow, H. (1923). *Brightness and dullness in children* (2nd ed.). Philadelphia: Lippincott.

Woolley, H. T., & Hart, H. (1921). Feeble-minded ex-school children: A study of children who have been students in Cincinnati special schools [Entire issue]. *Studies from the Helen S. Trounstine Foundation, 1* (7), 237–264.

Wormwald, J., & Wormwald, S. (1913). *A guide to the Mental Deficiency Act, 1913*. London: King & Son.

Wright, J. D. (1915). *What the mother of a deaf child ought to know*. New York: Stokes.

Yell, M. L., Rogers, D., & Rogers, E. L. (1998). The legal history of special education: What a long, strange trip it's been. *Remedial and Special Education, 19* (4), 219–228.

Young, M. (1916). *The mentally defective child*. London: Lewis.

Zedler, E. Y. (1953). Public opinion and public education for the exceptional child–court decisions 1873–1950. *Exceptional Children, 19* (5), 187–198.

Zook, G. F. (1934). Review and forecast. *School Life, 19*, 205.

Author Index

Subject Index